PRACTICAL PHARMACEUTICAL CHEMISTRY

PRACTICAL PHARMACEUTICAL CHEMISTRY

DR. ANEES AHMED SIDDIQUI
DR. MOHAMMED ALI
Faculty of Pharmacy
Jamia Hamdard
(Hamdard University)
Hamdard Nagar
New Delhi-110062

CBSPD

CBS Publishers & Distributors Pvt Ltd

New Delhi • Bengaluru • Chennai • Kochi • Kolkata • Lucknow • Mumbai
Hyderabad • Jharkhand • Nagpur • Patna • Pune • Uttarakhand

Practical Pharmaceutical Chemistry

ISBN: 978-81-239-0570-9

First Edition: 1997
Reprint: 2001, 2003, 2004, 2005, 2006, 2007, 2008, 2013, 2017, 2018, 2019, 2023

Published by **Satish Kumar Jain** and produced by **Varun Jain** for

CBS Publishers & Distributors Pvt Ltd

4819/XI Prahlad Street, 24 Ansari Road, Daryaganj, New Delhi 110 002, India.
Ph: 011-23289259, 23266861, 23266867 Website: www.cbspd.com
Fax: 011-23243014 e-mail: delhi@cbspd.com;

Corporate Office: 204 FIE, Industrial Area, Patparganj, Delhi 110 092
Ph: 011-4934 4934 Fax: 011-4934 4935 e-mail: publishing@cbspd.com; publicity@cbspd.com

Branches

- **Bengaluru:** Seema House 2975, 17th Cross, KR Road, Banasankari 2nd Stage, Bengaluru 560 070, Karnataka, India
  Ph: +91-80-26771678/79 Fax: +91-80-26771680 e-mail: bangalore@cbspd.com
- **Chennai:** 7, Subbaraya Street, Shenoy Nagar, Chennai 600 030, Tamil Nadu, India
  Ph: +91-44-26680620, 26681266 Fax: +91-44-42032115 e-mail: chennai@cbspd.com
- **Kochi:** 42/1325, 1326, Power House Road, Opp KSEB, Power House, Ernakulum Kochi 682 018, Kerala, India
  Ph: +91-484-4059061-65,67 Fax: +91-484-4059065 e-mail: kochi@cbspd.com
- **Kolkata:** 147, Hind Ceramics Compound, 1st Floor, Nilgunj Road, Belghoria, Kolkata-700056, West Bengal, India
  Ph: +033-25633055, 033-25633056 e-mail: kolkata@cbspd.com
- **Lucknow:** Basement, Khushnuma Complex, 7 Meerabai Marg (Behind Jawahar Bhawan),Lucknow-226001, UP, India
  Ph: +0522-4000032 e-mail: tiwari.lucknow@cbspd.com
- **Mumbai:** PWD Shed, Gala no 25/26, Ramchandra Bhatt Marg, Next to JJ Hospital Gate no. 2, Opp. Union Bank of India, Noorbaug, Mumbai-400009, Maharashtra, India
  Ph: 022-66661880/89 e-mail: mumbai@cbspd.com

Representatives

- Hyderabad 0-9885175004
- Jharkhand 0-9811541605
- Nagpur 0-9421945513
- Patna 0-9334159340
- Pune 0-9923910676
- Uttarakhand 0-9716462459

Printed at SRK Graphic, Shadara, Delhi

Preface

Practical part of every branch of science plays a very significant role since the basis of science is dependent on the verification of facts by experiment work. The practical aspect of pharmaceutical chemistry is concerned with the determination of physical constants, performance of colour tests, derivatization, synthesis, volumetric and gravimetric analyses, limit tests, etc. The present book is written to fulfil the requirements of undergraduate students of pharmacy course. The general format of presentation of each chapter includes introduction and experimental procedures. Chemical reactions are mentioned to make the subject simple and understandable.

A separate chapter for the preparation of reagents and solution is given. The methods of recording experiments of volumetric analysis and quantitative organic analysis are presented in the Appendix I and Appendix II, respectively. It is hoped that the book will satisfy all the requirements of students concerning chemistry practicals.

The authors wish to thank all the readers of previous textbooks who appreciated the compliments. We acknowledge a very pleasent and fruitful association with Shri Satish Kumar Jain and Vinod Kumar Jain, CBS Publishers & Distributors. The assignment could not have been completed without their encouragement and assistant. We are thankful to Shri Girendra Singh, Phoenix Computers, for typesetting the book on a laser printer and co-operating with us for extensive editing of the book several times.

We feel pleasure in expressing our sincere thanks to Mr. Mohd. Islam Ansari of our Faculty who has been associating with the chemistry practicals since last twenty years. He always felt a scarcity of a practical book of Pharmaceutical Chemistry and stressed us to compile the same at the earliest. We express our indebtedness to those authors of monographs, articles and books from which we have gained so much information for writing the manuscript. Our greatest debt of gratitude is due to our family members for sharing us to compile the book.

All constructive criticism and comments on the book from students and teachers are most welcome and shall form the basis for improving future editions.

Dr. Anees Ahmed Siddiqui
Dr. Mohammed Ali

Contents

1
Introduction

Apparatus and Basic Techniques

Before starting an experiment, cleaning of glassware, equipments and bench is necessary. The bench should be kept clean to remove any solid or liquid chemicals. Glassware are first washed with a detergent and then rinsed with distilled water before use. The outer surface may be dried with a cloth or filter paper. All the apparatus used in a particular experiment should be kept together on the bench to avoid confusion in determining the duplicate experiments. Excess of apparatus, which are not in use, should be removed from the bench. All the solutions, precipitates and filtrates should be labelled to avoid confusion and covered to prevent contamination of the contents. Reagent bottles must be returned on the reagent shelves immediately after use. Experimental observations must be recorded in a stiff covered note book containing an index page and remaining one-sided line pages. The record must be concluded with calculations and the results.

Glassware

The convenient unit to measure the large volume of a liquid is 'litre'. The litre and millilitre are sufficiently precise for the requirements of titrimetric analysis.

The capacity of a glass vessel varies with temperature. Therefore, the temperature of the experiment is noted.

Graduated Apparatus : Graduated flasks, burettes and pipettes are the most commonly used apparatus in volumetric analysis. All these glassware must be perfectly clean from grease to get exact results. Many detergents are available for cleaning the glass apparatus. Saturated solution of powdered sodium and potassium dichromate in concentrated sulphuric acid is also used for cleaning purpose.

Volumetric Flasks : A volumetric flask is a flat-bottomed, pear-shaped apparatus with long narrow neck. A thin line mark around the neck indicates the volume that it holds at a certain definite temperature, usually 20°C. The capacity and temperature are clearly marked on the flask. Both the front and the back of the mark should be seen as a single line to avoid errors due to parallax when making the final adjustment. The lower edge of the meniscus should be tangential to the graduation mark. A small change in the volume is detected easily in the long narrow neck.

Volumetric flasks are available in capacities of 1, 2, 5, 10, 20, 50, 100, 200, 250, 500, 1000, 2000, and 5000 cm^3. The standard solutions are obtained for analysis with the help of pipette.

Pipettes : Pipettes are of two type :

(i) *transfer pipettes*, which have one mark and withdraw a small and constant volume of the solution; (ii) *measuring or graduated pipettes*, which are graduated and used to deliver various small volumes.

The *transfer pipette* is made up of a cylindrical bulb joined at both ends to narrower tubing. A calibration mark is present around the upper tube while the lower delivery tube is made to a fine tip. This type of pipette is used to deliver pre-determined variable volumes of liquid. The transfer pipettes are constructed with capacities of 1, 2, 5, 10, 20, 25, 50 and 100 cm^3. The pipettes of the capacities of 10, 25 and 50 cm^3 are frequently used in macro work.

Before using, the pipettes are first rinsed with the liquid, then filled by suction to about 2-3 cm above the mark and the upper end of the pipette is closed with the tip of the finger. The liquid is allowed to run out slowly by slightly relaxing the pressure of the finger and rotating the pipette until the bottom of the meniscus just reached the graduation mark. The pipette is held vertically to fix the mark at the same level as the eye. The adhering drops at the tip are removed by stroking against a glass surface. The liquid is transferred into a flask keeping the tip of the pipette in contact with the wall of the flask. When all the solution is transferred, the upper end is closed with the tip of the finger and the cylindrical bulb is closed with fingers of the other hand to discharge the last drop of the jet. It may also be discharged by blowing.

Corrosive or toxic liquids are drawn in the pipette with the help of rubber or plastic bulb with glass ball valves operated between finger and thumb. A piston-control is also attached to the suction end of the pipette.

Graduated pipettes are made up of straight, narrow tubes with no central bulbs. They deliver a measured volume from a top zero to a selected graduation mark or to the jet, i.e. the zero is at the set.

Burettes : Burettes are long cylindrical tubes with uniform bore throughout the graduated length, a narrow lower end with a glass stopcock and a jet. When in use, a burette must be firmly supported on a stand with a burette holder. The stopcock should be lubricated to prevent sticking or freezing and ensure smoothness in action. Vaseline may be used as a lubricant.

Before using, the burette is thoroughly cleaned with a cleaning agent, rinsed well with distilled water, the stopcock is lubricated and fixed in a burette holder. The solution is filled with the help of a small funnel up to zero mark. The liquid is discharged from a burette into a conical flask. The flask is gently rotated with the right hand for mixing the contents well.

Purified water : Purified distilled water is used in analytical operations. Highly pure water is obtained by allowing tap water to percolate through a mixture of ion-exchange resins. A strong acid resin will remove cations from the water and replace them by hydrogen ions, and a strong base resin will remove anions by hydroxyl ions. Various commercial units are available for the preparation of de-ionized water.

Wash-bottles : A wash-bottle is a flat-bottomed flask fitted up to withdraw a fine stream of distilled water. The thumb is kept over the tube and water is blown out.

A polythene wash bottle is cheap, fitted with a plastic cap and a plastic jet and has flexible sides. Pressure is applied by squeezing and jet of water is controlled.

Filtration apparatus : A conical funnel fitted with a filter paper is usually used for filtration. The funnel should have an angle nearly 60° and a long stem.

Sintered glass crucibles are made of resistance glass and have porous disc fused into the body of the crucible. The filter disc is made up of various pore diameters as indicated by numbers from 0 to 5.

Buchner funnel is used to filter large quantities of material. A good quality of filter paper is placed on the plate. With sintered glass plate no filter paper is needed.

2

Titrimetric Analysis

Titrimetric analysis is the quantitative chemical analysis which is performed by determining the volume of a solution of accurately known concentration required to react quantitatively with the solution of the substance to be determined. The solution of accurately known strength is called the **standard solution** which is taken in a burette. The process of addition of the standard solution until the reaction is just complete is called a **titration**, and the substance to be determined is **titrant.** The point at which this reaction is completed is called the **equivalent point** or **end point** which is detected by the addition of an **indicator**. On completion of the reaction, the indicator should give a clear visual change in the liquid being titrated.

Standard Solutions : A standard solution contains a known weight of the reagent in a definite volume of solution; the concentration is expressed as mole.

The mole is the amount of substances which contains as many elementary units as there are atoms in 0.012 kilogram of carbon 12. It is termed as gram-molecule, gram-ion, etc.

Molarity : A molar solution is one which contains the gram-molecular weight of a substance in one litre of solution. The strengths of molar solutions are independent of the reaction. It is designated as M.

Normality : A normal solution (expressed as N) is a solution which contains one gram equivalent of substance per litre of solution. The strengths of the solutions are designated as: twice normal (2 N), half normal (0.5 or N/2), decinormal (0.1 N or N/10) and centi-normal (0.01 N or N/100).

Equivalent Weight: The equivalent weight of an acid or base is that weight of it which contains 1.008 g of replaceable hydrogen or its equivalent, such as hydroxyl group. The equivalent weights of hydrochloric acid (HCl) and sodium hydroxide (NaOH) are equal of their molecular weights.

Sulphuric acid (H_2SO_4) and oxalic acid (COOH-COOH) contain two replaceable hydrogens, therefore, their equivalent weights are equal to half the respective molecular weights.

The equivalent of a base is that mass of it which contains one replaceable hydroxyl group, i.e. 17.008 g of equivalent to 1.008 g of hydrogen. The equivalents of sodium hydroxide and potassium hydroxide are the mole (1 N); calcium hydroxide and barium hydroxide are half a mole (0.5 N).

In oxidation-reduction titrations, the equivalent weight is that weight which combines with 1.008 g of available hydrogen or 8.000 g of available oxygen for use in the oxidation or reduction reaction under consideration.

In precipitation reaction, as in argentimetry, the equivalent weight is defined as that weight of substance which contains or combines with 1 g atom or a univalent metal.

Calculation of Equivalent Weight

Hydrochloric Acid $HCl \equiv H$

Therefore, $(1+35.45) = 36.45\ HCl \equiv 1000$ ml N

Sodium Carbonate

$$Na_2CO_3 + 2HCl \longrightarrow 2NaCl + H_2O + CO_2$$

Therefore, $Na_2CO_3 \equiv 2HCl \equiv 2H$

$(2 \times 23 + 12 + 3 \times 16) = 106$ g of $Na_2CO_3 \equiv 2000$ ml N HCl.

or 53 g $Na_2CO_3 \equiv 1000$ ml N HCl

Sodium Acid Oxalate

The equivalent weight varies with the reaction under consideration :

1. As a Neutralizing Agent

$$NaHC_2O_4 + NaOH \longrightarrow Na_2C_2O_4 + H_2O$$

Therefore, $NaHC_2O_4 \equiv NaOH \equiv H$

$(23 + 1 + 24 + 64) = 112$ g of $NaHC_2O_4 \equiv 1000$ ml N NaOH

2. As a Reducing Agent

$$NaHC_2O_4 + O \longrightarrow NaOH + 2CO_2$$

Therefore, $NaHC_2O_4 \equiv O \equiv 2H$

$(23 + 1 + 24 + 64) = 112$ g $NaHC_2O_4 \equiv 2000$ ml N

or 56 g $NaHC_2O_4 \equiv 1000$ ml N NaOH

Equivalence of Standard Solutions

If an acid A of volume v_A is titrated to neutrality against a base of volume v_B, then since the two solutions contain the same number of gram equivalents,

$$v_A \times \text{normality}_A = v_B \times \text{normality}_B$$

If the normality of one solution is known, the equivalent volumes of two solutions are determined by titration, and the normality of the second solution can be found out.

Preparation of Standard Solution

If the chemical compound is available in a pure state, an exact equivalent amount is weighed, dissolved in water and made up to volume. The compounds, which are not obtained in pure state, e.g. caustic soda, mineral acids, are prepared a little more concentrated than are required, and to dilute it with distilled water until the desired normality is obtained. The solutions must be standardized. The compounds available in highly pure form and suitable for the preparation of standard solutions are sodium carbonate, sodium tetraborate, sodium oxalate, sodium chloride, potassium chloride, potassium bromate, potassium iodate, potassium dichromate, arsenic (III) oxide, benzoic acid, and potassium hydrogen phthalate.

When the reagent is not available in the pure form, e.g. most alkali solutions, some inorganic acids, deliquescent substances, etc., solutions of the approximate normality required are first prepared. These solution are then standardized by titration against a solution of a pure substance of known concentration.

Table 1 : Equivalent Weights of Some Acids and Bases

Compound	Molecular weight	Acidity/ Basicity/loss or gain of electrons	Equivalent weight
Hydrochloric acid	36.46	1	36.46
Nitric acid	63.01	1	63.01
Sulphuric acid	98.07	2	49.03
Acetic acid	60.05	1	60.05
Boric acid	61.83	3	20.61
Sodium hydroxide	40.0	1	40.00
Potassium hydroxide	56.11	1	56.11
Sodium carbonate	105.99	2	53.00
Sodium bicarbonate	84.01	1	84.01
Potassium carbonate	138.21	2	69.10
Potassium bicarbonate	100.12	1	100.12
Potassium permanganate	158.03	5	31.60
Potassium dichromate	294.18	6	49.03
Iodine	253.8	2	126.90
Oxalic acid (anhydrous)	90.0	2	45.00
Oxalic acid (dihydrate)	126.07	2	63.03
Ferrous sulphate (anhydrous)	152.0	1	152.00
Ferrous sulphate (heptahydrate)	278.0	1	278.00
Ferrous ammonium sulphate	392.13	1	392.13
Sodium thiosulphate (pentahydrate)	248.17	1	248.17

Factors : The standard solutions are only approximately N, 0.5 N and 0.1, etc. The relationship of the exact strength of such a solution to the nominal normality of the solution is then indicated by a factor, defined as the number of millilitres of exactly N, 0.5 N, etc. solutions which are equivalent to 1 ml of the solution of the same nominal normality. It is the number by which the actual volume of the solution of approximate strength must be multiplied to obtain the equivalent volume of a standard solution of exact normality.

Factor in Standardization of N H_2SO_4 by N Na_2CO_3

If 20 ml N Na_2CO_3 is neutralized by 19.40 ml of N H_2SO_4,

Then, 19.40 ml of $H_2SO_4 \equiv$ 20 ml N Na_2CO_3

$$\text{Therefore, 1 ml N } H_2SO_4 \equiv \frac{20}{19.40} \text{ ml N} \equiv 1.031 \text{ ml N}$$

Therefore, the strength of the H_2SO_4 solution is N (1.031). The factor of the solution is 1.031 and all volumes of this solution when multiplies by 1.031 will be the equipment volume of normal solution.

Reactions in Titrimetric Analysis

Two types of reactions are involved in titrimetric analysis:

1. Those in which there is no change in oxidation state; these are dependent upon the combination of ions.

2. Oxidation-reduction reactions in which a change of oxidation state is involved.

Generally, these two types of reactions are divided into four main classes;

1. *Acidimetry and alkalimetry or Neutralization reaction*
2. *Complex formation reactions*
3. *Precipitation reactions*
4. *Oxidation-reduction reactions*

Acidimetry and Alkalimetry or Neutralization reaction

A neutralization reaction involves the titration of free bases with a standard acid (*acidimetry*), and the titration of free acid with a base (*alkalimetry*). These reactions include the combination of hydrogen and hydroxide ion to form water. The point at which this is reached is the equivalence point or theoretical end-point. If both the acid and base are strong electrolytes, the resultant solution will be neutral and have a pH of 7. If either the acid or the base is a weak electrolyte, the salt will be hydrolyzed to some extent and the solution at the equivalence point will be either slightly alkaline or slightly acid.

The acid-base indicators possess different colours according to the hydrogen-ion concentration of the solution, and the position of the colour-change interval in the pH scale varies widely with different indicators.

In aqueous solution an acid is dissociated into hydrogen ion and anion (Cl^-, HSO_4^-, NO_3^-, etc.).

$$HCl \rightleftharpoons H^+ + Cl^- \rightleftharpoons H_3O^+$$

The hydrogen ion combines with water to give hydronium ion (H_3O^+).

An alkali on dissociation in water gives hydroxyl ions,

$$NaOH \rightleftharpoons Na^+ + OH^-$$

The neutralization reaction is the reaction between an acid and a base to give a salt.

$$HCl + NaOH \longrightarrow NaCl + H_2O$$

Preparation of Indicator Solutions: If a substance, like sodium salts, is soluble in water, it is dissolved in water. In most cases 70—90 % ethanol is used.

Methyl Orange : Dissolve 0.5 g of methyl orange (free acid) in 1 litre of water and filter, if necessary. When methyl orange is in the salt form, dissolve 0.5 g of the sodium salt in 1 litre of water, add 15.2 ml of 0.1 M, HCl and filter, if necessary.

Methyl Red : Dissolve 1 g of the free acid in 1 litre of hot water or in 600 ml of ethanol and dilute with 400 ml of water.

Phenolphthalein : Dissolve 5 g of the reagent in 500 ml of ethanol and add 500 ml of water with constant stirring. If a precipitate is formed, filter it.

Thymolphthalein : Dissolve 0.4 g of the reagent in 600 ml of ethanol and add 400 ml of water with stirring.

1–Naphthalein : Dissolve 0.1 g of the indicator in 500 ml of ethanol and dilute with 500 ml of water.

Quinaldine Red : Dissolve 1 g in 100 ml of 80% ethanol.

Methyl Yellow, Neutral Red, and Congo Red : Dissolve 1 g of the indicator in 1 litre of 80% ethanol. Congo red may also be dissolved in water.

4–Nitrophenol : Dissolve 2 g of the solid in 1 litre of water.

Alizarin Yellow R : Dissolved 0.5 g of the indicator in 1 litre of 80% ethanol.

Tropaeolin : Dissolve 1 g of the solid in 1 litre of water.

Mixed Indicators : Mixed indicators are used to get sharp colour change over a narrow and selected range of pH by the use of a suitable mixture of indicators. For example, a mixture of equal parts of neutral red (0.1% in ethanol) and methylene blue (0.1% in ethanol) gives a sharp colour change from violet-blue to green at pH 7. This indicator is used in the titration of acetic acid with ammonia solution or vice versa. A mixture of phenolphthalein (3 parts of a 0.1% aqueous solution of the sodium salt) and cresol red (1 part of a 0.1% aqueous solution of the sodium salt) changes from yellow to violet at pH 8.3 and is recommended for the titration of carbonate to the hydrogen-carbonate stage.

Standardization of N H_2SO_4 : The reaction involved in the titration of sulphuric acid with sodium carbonate, is

$$H_2SO_4 + Na_2CO_3 \longrightarrow Na_2SO_4 + CO_2 + H_2O$$

Procedure : Heat sodium carbonate in a nickel crucible at 260—270° for 30 minutes to remove any trace of water. Cool in a desiccator, weigh, dissolve in a graduated flask containing water, dilute to volume and mix thoroughly. Pipette 20 ml of this solution into a conical flask, add methyl orange indicator (1 drop) and titrate with the sulphuric acid solution to get orange colour. Repeat with another 20 ml portion. The two titrations should be within 0.05 ml.

This method can be applied to the standardization of other strengths of acid solutions.

Standardization of N NaOH

Solutions of sodium hydroxide are always standardized by titration with standard acids of equivalent normality. They always contain a small amount of carbon dioxide fixed as sodium carbonate and must be considered when standardizing alkali hydroxide solutions:

$$NaOH + HCl \longrightarrow NaCl + H_2O$$

$$Na_2CO_3 + HCl \longrightarrow NaHCO_3 + NaCl$$

$$NaHCO_3 + HCl \longrightarrow NaCl + H_2CO_3$$

$$\downarrow$$

$$CO_2 + H_2O$$

The hydrochloric acid is run into the sodium hydroxide solution. Several end points of these reactions can be determined by suitable choice of indicators. Phenolphthalein is sensitive to carbon dioxide and gives pink colour with the indicator. Methyl orange end point is obtained.

Procedure : Pipette 20 ml of 1 N NaOH into a conical flask, add 2 drops of phenolphthalein solution, and titrate with N HCl until the solution is just colourless. Note the burette reading for calculation of the phenolphthalein factor, add 1 drop of methyl orange solution, and continue the titration until the first orange colour is obtained. Record the burette reading and calculate the methyl orange factor. The standardization should be carried out in duplicate.

Titration of Strong Acids

Titration of strong acids with sodium hydroxide solution gives salts which are not hydrolyzed in aqueous solution. The solution becomes neutral at the equivalence point. The pH changes extremely rapidly in the region of the equivalent point, and an indicator, which changes colour within the range between pH 4 and 10, is suitable. Methyl orange is generally used for such titrations.

$$\underset{36.46}{HCl} + \underset{40}{NaOH} \longrightarrow \underset{58.46}{NaCl} + \underset{18}{H_2O}$$

Therefore, 36.46 g of HCl ≡ 40 g of NaOH

or 1 g equivalent of HCl ≡ 1 g equivalent of NaOH

When 1000 ml of 1 N solution of NaOH is mixed with 1000 ml of 1 N solution of HCl, the two substances react in their equal equivalents.

If V_1 ml of solution of NaOH of N_1 normality, the number of gram-equivalent can be determined as :

$$\text{normality} = \frac{\text{Number of gram equivalents}}{\text{Volume in litres}}$$

or number of gram equivalent = normality × volume in litres.

Therefore, the number of gram equivalents of NaOH in solution of volume V_1 ml of N_1 normality is

$$= \frac{N_1 \times V_1}{1000}$$

The number of gram equivalents of HCl in volume V_2 ml of N_2 normality is = $\frac{N_2 \times V_2}{1000}$

The gram-equivalents of NaOH react with equal gram equivalents of HCl on completion of neutralization,

$$\frac{N_1 \times V_1}{1000} = \frac{N_2 \times V_2}{1000}$$

or

$$N_1V_2 = N_2V_2$$

This normality equation is used to calculate the normality of the unknown solution. If the volumes V_1, V_2 and the normality N_1 are known, the normality N_2 can be calculated.

For determining the percentage purity, a known weight of the substance is dissolved in definite volume of water. By titrating this solution with a suitable titrant, the normality of the solution is found out. By multiplying the normality with the equivalent weight of the solute, its strength in grams per litre is determined.

$$\text{Purity of the substance in percentage} = \frac{\text{Grams per litre of substance calculated after titration}}{\text{Grams per litre of the substance dissolved}}$$

Complexometric Titrations

A complexation reaction with a metal ion involves the replacement of one or more of the co-ordinated solvent molecules by other nucleophilic groups. A complexing agent is any electron-donationg ion or molecule, called *ligand*, which produces one or more covalent bonds with the metal ions and forms a complex which has different properties from those of the free metal ions. Complex formation takes place in the titration of a solution of a cyanide with silver nitrate or of chloride ion with mercury (II) nitrate solution.

$$2CN + Ag^+ \rightleftharpoons [Ag(CN)_2]^-$$

$$2Cl + Hg^{2+} \rightleftharpoons HgCl_2$$

The complexing agent holds a metal ion in complex through one or more co-ordinate or covalent bonds. There is a specific number of ligands that are bound to each metal ion. This is based on a specific co-ordination number which varies for each metal ion. A metal ion has more than one co-ordination number. The ferricyanide ion may be consisted of three ordinary covalent and three co-ordinate bonds. In a complex the bonds are identical hybrid bonds which are directed towards the apices of a regular octahedron.

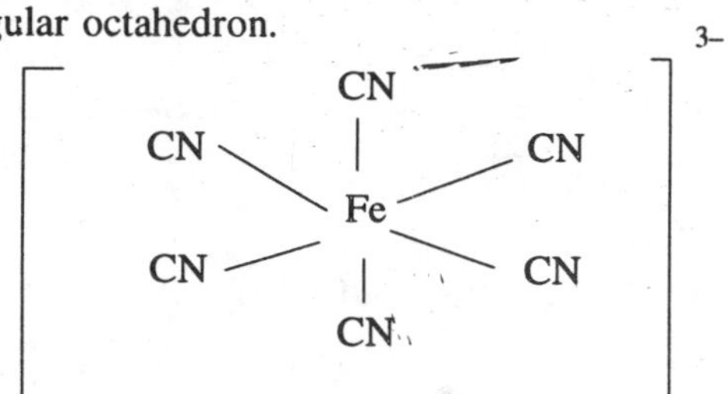

Hybrid bonds

Complexes involving simple ligands forming only one bond are called *co-ordination compounds*. Ligands having two or more electron-donating groups are known as *chelating agents* forming cyclic structures. 1,2-Diaminoethane behaves like two ammonia molecules and forms *chelates* with copper and cobalt ions.

Organic compounds containing groups with an easily replaceable proton (–COOH, phenolic OH) or neutral groups having a lone pair of electrons (NH_2, CO, alcoholic OH) form chelates. The greater the number of rings which can be formed, the more stable will be the chelates. The solubility of metal chelates in water depends upon the presence of hydrophilic groups such as COOH, SO_3H, NH_2 and OH. When both acidic and basic groups are present, the complex will be soluble over a wide range of pH.

Ethylenediaminetetraacetic acid, EDTA, is a very important reagent for complex formation titration. Dimethylglyoxime and salicyladoxime are chelating agents, forming insoluble complexes. EDTA reacts with most polyvalent metal ions to form water-soluble complexes which cannot be extracted from aqueous solution with organic solvents. Dimethylglyoxime and salicylaldoxime form water-insoluble complexes which are soluble in organic solvents.

Complexes of most divalent metals are stable in ammonical solution. Trivalent metal complexes are usually still more firmly bound and stable in strongly acid solutions. For example, the cobalt (Co^{3+}) edetate complex is stable in concentrated hydrochloric acid. Increase in temperature causes a slight increase in the ionization of the complex and a slight lowering of stability constant.

Colour of Complexes : There is a change in the absorption spectrum when complexes are formed which is a basis of many colorimetric assays.

Titration of Metal Ions using Disodium Edetate : Edetic acid is sparingly soluble in water. Edetate solution is run into a solution of a metal ion buffered to promote efficient complex formation. The end point of complexometric titrations is shown by means of *pM indicator* which is a dye capable of acting as a chelating agent to give a dye-metal complex. The dye-metal complex is different in colour from the dye itself. When there is the slightest excess of edetate, the metal-dye complex decomposes to produce free dye, this is accomplished by a change in colour.

In complexometric titrations, a metal-ion indicator shows the colour due to the dye-metal complex until the end point when an equivalent amount of EDTA titrant has been added. When there is a slight excess of EDTA titrant, the dye-metal complex decomposes to form free dye and there is a change in colour which is dependent on pH of the solution. The pH variation also affects the stability of the complex. Therefore, a buffer solution is used to maintain the required pH during the titration.

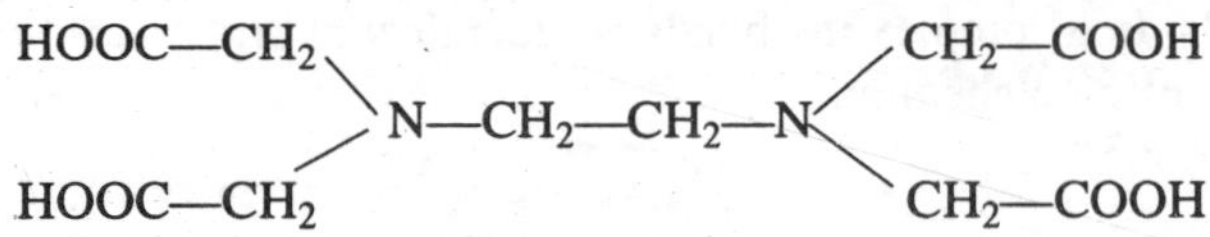

EDTA

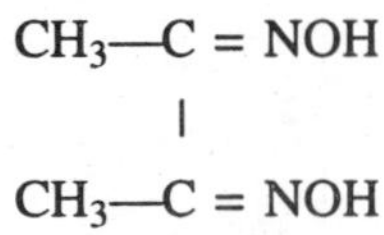

Dimethylglyoxime

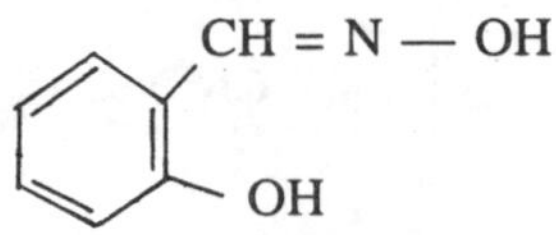

Salicylaldoxime

pM Indicators

Murexide

Murexide is ammonium purpurate which is used for the titration of calcium at pH 12. Calcium is bound in an eight – membered ring in the murexide chelate which is less stable in comparison to five – and six – membered ring chelates. Since magnesium – murexide in less stable then the calcium complex, calcium is titrated in the presence of magnesium as in water analysis.

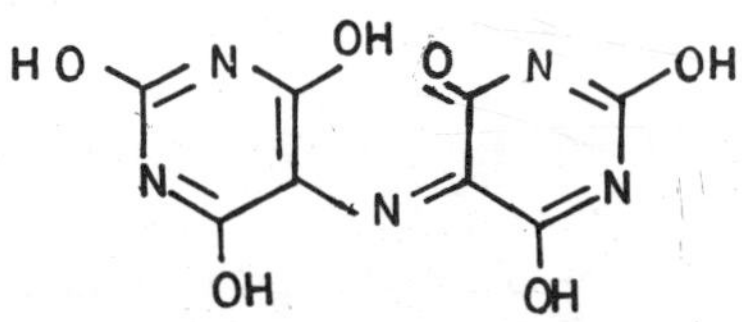

.Murexide (violet at pH 12)

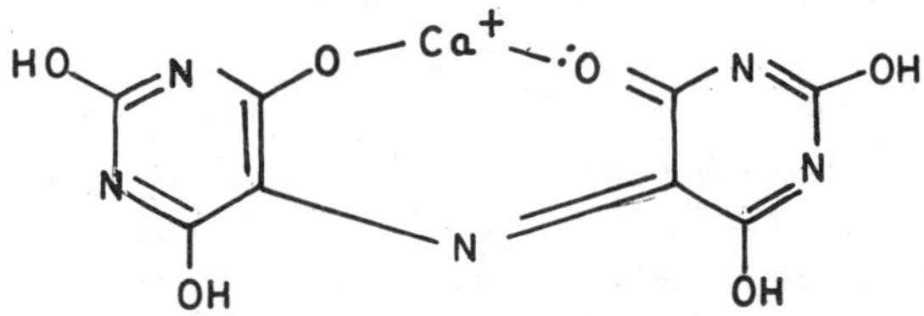

Calcium murexide complex

Copper, cobalt and cerium form yellow complexes with murexide in alkaline solution. They give clear colour changes when titrated with sodium edetate.

Mordant Black 2 (Eriochrome Black T).

This indicator is blue at about pH 10 and most of its complexes are reddish. Below pH 6.3 and above pH 11.5, the dye itself is reddish. The titration is carried out in the presence of a buffer at pH 10.

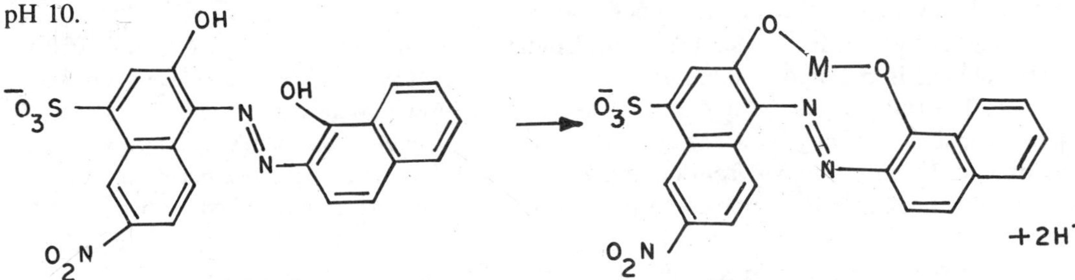

Blue (pH 10) Pink

Magnesium, calcium, cadmium, zinc, manganese, lead and mercury are titrated directly using this indicator. Cobalt, nickel, copper, aluminium, silver, titanium and platinum form more stable complexes with the dye than with the edetate. Therefore, the dye cannot be used as an indicator.

Catechol Violet

The catechols form weak, highly-coloured complexes in neutral, acid and alkaline solutions.

All the complexes are blue in alkaline solution. In this solution, clear end points are shown with magnesium, manganese, iron, cobalt, nickel, zinc, cadmium and calcium.

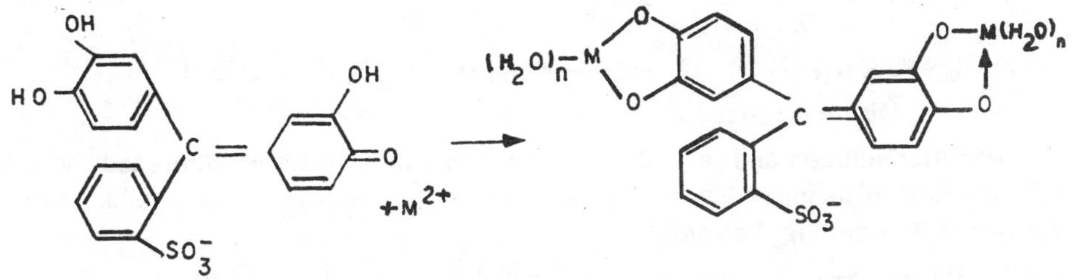

Blue (pH 10) Pink

Xylenol Orange : This is an acid-base indicator having the same characteristics as cresol red. It is used to titrate metals whose edetate complexes are stable in acid solution, e.g. bismuth, thorium, lead, lanthanum, cadmium and mercury. The stability of the complexes varies with pH.

Methyl Thymol Blue : It is derived from thymol blue and used for bismuth in strongly acid solution and for lead, zinc, cadmium, mercury and cobalt in weakly acid solution.

Alizarin Fluorine Blue : It is used in acid solution at pH 4.3 for the titration of lead, zinc, cobalt (Co^{2+}), mercury (Hg^{2+}) and copper (Cu^{2+}) when the colour changes from red to yellow. It is also used in the determination of fluorine in some synthetic drugs.

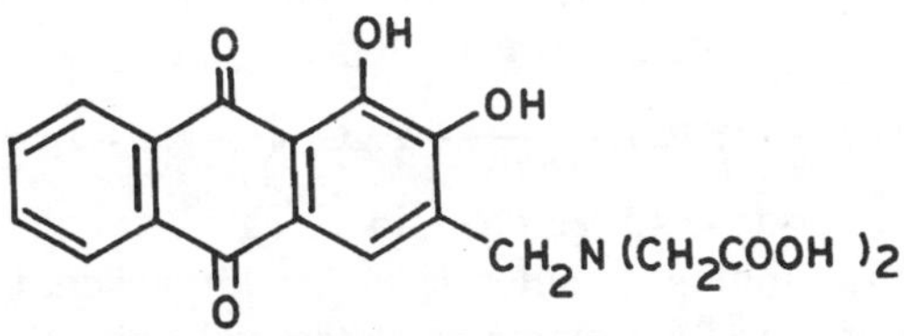

Sodium Alizarinesulphonate : It yields a bluish-red colour with aluminium and thorium ions at pH 4 and a yellow in the absence of these ions. It is used to determine fluorine in Triamcinolone by titration with standard thorium nitrate solution.

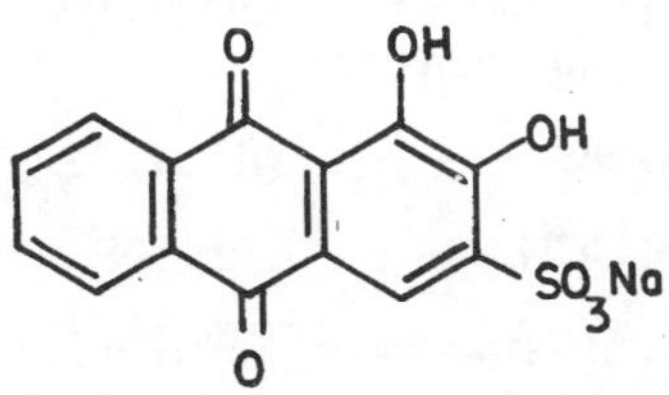

Diphenylcarbazone is used an indicator for determination of mercury in methylthiouracil. *Tiron* forms a blue colour with ferric iron between pH 2 and 5, a violet colour between pH 5.7 and 7 and a red complex in alkaline solution.

$C_6H_5N = NCONHC_6H_5$

Diphenyl carbazone

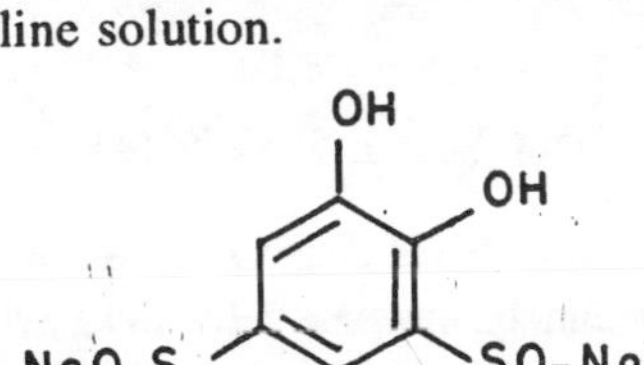

Tiron

Standardization : Preparation and standardization of 0.05M disodium edetate solution is based on titration of the prepared disodium edetate solution with a standard zinc chloride solution prepared from a known weight of granulated zinc.

$$Zn + 2HCl \longrightarrow ZnCl_2 + H_2$$

$$\underset{\text{Disodium edetate}}{ZnCl_2 + C_{10}H_{14}N_2Na_2O_8} \longrightarrow C_{10}H_{14}N_2O_8Zn + 2NaCl$$

A suitable buffer solution and indicator are added to the metal ion solution and the solution titrated with standard disodium edetate until the indicator just changes colour. A blank tritration may be performed by omitting the sample.

Dissolve disodium edetate (18.61g) in sufficient amount of water to produce 1000 ml. Mordant black 11 mixture is used as an indicator in ammonia buffer.

Dissolve granulated zinc (0.8g) in dilute hydrochloric acid (12 ml) and bromine water (0.1 ml) by gentle warming. Boil to remove excess of bromine, cool and add sufficient water to produce 200 ml. Pipette 20 ml of the resulting solution into a flask and neutralize with 2M sodium hydroxide solution. Dilute the solution with water (150 ml), add sufficient buffer (pH 10.0) to dissolve edetate solution until the solution turns green.

Factor : Each ml of 0.05 M disodium edetate is equivalent to 0.000654 g of zinc.

PRECIPITATION METHODS

It involves the formation of precipitation by the titrants as in silver nitrate titration.

Silver Nitrate Titration : When silver nitrate solution is run into a solution of sodium chloride, a precipitate of silver chloride is formed:

$$NaCl + AgNO_3 \longrightarrow AgCl\downarrow + NaNO_3$$

At the end point all the chloride has been precipitated as silver chloride. Potassium chromate is used as an indicator in the titration of chloride ions with standard silver nitrate in neutral solution, giving a precipitate of red silver chromate at the end point. Ferric alum is used as an indicator for the titration of silver ions with ammonium thiocyanate solution in the presence of nitric acid. When excess of standard silver nitrate solution is added to a solution of the halide, precipitation of silver halide occurs. The excess of silver nitrate is then back titrated with ammonium thiocyanate. At the end point, excess of thiocyanate reacts with ferric ions to give red colour due to formation of ferric ferrithiocyanate:

$$MX + AgNO_3 \longrightarrow MNO_3 + AgX\downarrow$$

$$AgNO_3 + NH_4SCN \longrightarrow AgSCN\downarrow + NH_4NO_3$$

$$2Fe^{3+} + 6SCN^- \rightleftharpoons \underset{\text{(Red Colour)}}{Fe^{3+}[Fe(SCN)_6]^{3-}}$$

In the determination of a chloride, the following equation is considered :

$$Ag^+ + Cl^- \rightleftharpoons AgCl\downarrow$$

$$Ag^+ + SCN^- \rightleftharpoons AgSCN\downarrow$$

Preparation and standardization of 0.1N $AgNO_3$ solution : AR Silver nitrate contains 99.9 to 100% $AgNO_3$. A 0.1 N solution can be prepared by dissolving 16.789 g of silver nitrate in water and adjusting to 1000 ml. A solution may be standardized against a standard solution of sodium chloride using potassium chromate as an indicator (Mohr's method).

The standardization depends upon the reactions expressed as follows:

$$AgNO_3 + NaCl \longrightarrow AgCl\downarrow + NaNO_3$$

$$AgNO_3 \equiv NaCl \equiv H$$

$$169.89 \text{ g } AgNO_3 \equiv 58.45 \text{ g NaCl} \equiv 1000 \text{ ml N}$$

Therefore, $0.01699 \text{ g } AgNO_3 \equiv 0.005845 \text{ g NaCl} \equiv 1 \text{ ml } 0.1 \text{ N } AgNO_3$

OXIDATION-REDUCTION TITRATIONS

Oxidation and reduction can be defined in terms of loss or gain of electrons. It may also be defined as that mass of the reagent which reacts with or contains 1.008 g available hydrogen or 8.000 g of available oxygen. The amount of available oxygen may be shown by the following equation:

$$2KMnO_4 \longrightarrow K_2O + 2MnO + 5O$$

In acid solution $2KMnO_4$ gives up 5 atoms of available oxygen, which is taken up by the reducing agent. Therefore, its equivalent is 2 $KMnO_4/10$. For potassium dichromate in acid solution, the equation is written as:

$$K_2 Cr_2 O_7 \longrightarrow K_2O + Cr_2 O_3 + 3O$$

The equivalent is $K_2 Cr_2 O_7/6$.

The oxidation of iron (II) chloride in aqueous solution takes place as:

$$2FeCl_2 + Cl_2 \longrightarrow 2FeCl_3 \quad \text{or} \quad 2Fe^{2+} + Cl_2 \longrightarrow 2Fe^{3+} + 2Cl^-$$

The ion Fe^{2+} is converted into ion Fe^{3+} (oxidation), and the neutral chlorine molecule into negatively charged chloride ion Cl^- (reduction). The conversion of Fe^{2+} into Fe^{3+} loses one electron and the change of the neutral chlorine molecule into chloride ions requires two electrons. Therefore, oxidation is a process involving a loss of electron, i.e.

$$Fe^{2+} - e^- = Fe^{3+} \text{ (oxidation)},$$

and the reduction is the process involving gain of electrons, i.e.

$$Cl_2 + 2e^- = 2Cl^- \text{ (Reduction)}$$

Therefore, *oxidation* is the process which involves the loss of one or more electrons by atoms or ions. *Reduction* is the process which results in the gain of one or more electrons by atoms or ions. An *oxidizing agent* is one that gains electrons and is reduced; a reducing agent is one that loses electrons and is oxidized, The oxidation-reduction processes are also known as *redox* processes.

Equivalent Weights : The equivalent weight of an oxidizing agent is the weight of the substance which reacts with or contains 1.008 g of available hydrogen or 8.000 g of available oxygen. It may also be defined as the weight which gains electrons equivalent of 1 faraday and can be determined by dividing the gram-molecular weight by the number of electrons gained by each molecule. The equivalent weight of a reducing agent is that weight which loses electrons equivalent to 1 faraday and is found out by dividing the gram-molecular weight by the number of electrons lost by each molecule.

Potassium permanganate acts as an oxidizing agent in acidified solution and releases 5 atoms of available oxygen which are utilized by a reducing agent. The equivalent of $KMnO_4$ is calculated as follows:

$$2KMnO_4 + 3H_2SO_4 \longrightarrow K_2SO_4 + 2MnSO_4 + 3H_2O + 5[O].$$

$$2KMnO_4 \equiv 5[O]$$

$$2 \times 158 \equiv 5 \times 16$$

Equivalent weight of $KMnO_4 = \frac{2 \times 158}{5 \times 16} = 31.6$

In a redox process permanganate ion is converted to manganous ion by the gain of 5 electrons. Therefore, its equivalent weight in one-fifth of its molecular weight, 158/5 = 31.6

$$MnO_4^- + 8H^+ + 5e^- \longrightarrow Mn^{2+} + 4H_2O$$

Two thiosulphate ($S_2O_3{}^{2-}$) ions are transformed to tetrathionate ($S_2O_6{}^{2-}$) ion in the redox reaction by the loss of two electrons. Therefore, the equivalent weight of sodium thiosulphate ($Na_2S_2O_3.5H_2O$) is equal to its molecular weight, 248.17.

$$2S_2O_3^{2-} \longrightarrow S_4O_6^{2-} + 2e^-$$

Acidified $KMnO_4$ oxidizes oxalic acid to carbon dioxide. In other words the oxalate ion is oxidized to carbon dioxide by the loss of two electrons.

$$HOOC-COOH.2H_2O + [O] \longrightarrow 2CO_2 + 3H_2O$$

The equivalent of oxalic acid is half its molecular weight, 126.07/2 = 63.035.

Indicators : The oxidized or reduced form acts as a self-indicator. Acidified solution of $KMnO_4$ has deep purple colour. A permanent pink colour is appeared at the end point when $KMnO_4$ is used as titrant. Ceric sulphate (yellow) and iodine (brown) are reduced to colourless ions at the end point.

Potassium ferricyanide is used as an external indicator in the titration of ferrous iron by potassium dichromate which gives a deep prussian blue colour with potassium ferricyanide due to the presence of ferrous ions. At the end point, ferric iron only is present and this does not give a colour with potassium ferricyanide.

In the standardization of sodium thiosulphate, iodine is liberated. Therefore, starch mucilage is used as an indicator. Starch combines with iodine to form a blue colour.

Diphenylamine, sodium diphenylaminosulphonate, diphenylbenzidine and ferroin are also used as indicators in redox titration.

Potassium Permanganate Solution

Potassium permanganate is used as an oxidizing substance as indicated by the following equation:

$$MnO_4^- + 8H^+ + 5e^- \longrightarrow Mn^{2+} + 4H_2O$$

Therefore, $KMnO_4 \equiv 5e^-$

158.0 g $KMnO_4 \equiv$ 5000 ml N

3.160 g $KMnO_4 \equiv$ 1000 ml 0.1 N $KMnO_4$

Preparation of 0.1N of $KMnO_4$ Solution : As potassium permanganate may contain a trace amount of manganese dioxide, volumetric solutions must be standardized.

Weigh about 3.2 g of $KMnO_4$, transfer to a 250 ml beaker containing cold water and stir thoroughly breaking up the crystals with a glass rod. Decant the solution through a small plug of glass wool in a funnel into a 1 litre graduated flask. Add more water to the beaker and repeat the process. Make the solution up to the graduation mark and mix by shaking well.

Standardization of 0.1 N $KMnO_4$ by Oxalic Acid

$$HOOC-COOH \longrightarrow 2CO_2 + 2H^+ + 2e^-$$

Therefore, $H_2C_2O_4.2H_2O \equiv 2e^-$

6.302 g $H_2C_2O_4.2H_2O \equiv$ 1000 ml 0.1 N $KMnO_4$

Procedure : Weigh accurately 6.3 g of oxalic acid, transfer into 1 litre graduated flask, dissolve in water and make up to the volume. Pipette out 20 ml of this solution, add concentrated sulphuric acid (about 5 ml) and warm to about 70°. Add the $KMnO_4$ solution from the burette. The first few drops result in a pink colour persisting for about 20 seconds. Wait until the colour disappears and then continue the titration in the usual manner. The end point is reached when a faint pink colour persists for about 30 seconds upon shaking the flask.

Note : Formation of a brown colour during the titration is caused by insufficient acid, using too high temperature or by the use of a dirty flask.

Titration of Iodine

In the titration of iodine in aqueous solution, the following reaction involves :

$$I_2 + 2e^- \longrightarrow 2\,I^-$$

Therefore, $I_2 = 2e^-$

$$126.9 \text{ g } I_2 \equiv 1000 \text{ ml N}$$

$$12.69 \text{ g } I_2 \equiv 1000 \text{ ml } 0.1 \text{ N iodine.}$$

Iodine is practically insoluble in water. It dissolves in solutions of potassium iodide due to polyiodide formation, KI_3, which behaves in solution as free iodine.

Preparation of 0.1 N Iodine Solution : Weigh about 3.2 g of iodine and transfer to a beaker containing potassium iodide (7.5 g) and water (10 ml). Dissolve, transfer to a 250 ml graduated flask and adjust to volume.

Note : Iodine is volatile and standard solutions should be stored in tightly stoppered glass bottles.

Standardization of 0.1 N Iodine Solution by Arsenic trioxide

In this standardization the following equation takes place :

$$As_2O_3 + 2H_2O \longrightarrow As_2O_5 + 4H^+ + 4e^-$$

Therefore, $As_2O_3 \equiv 4e^-$

$$197.8 \text{ g } As_2O_3 \equiv 4000 \text{ ml N}$$

$$0.4946 \text{ g } As_2O_3 \equiv 100 \text{ ml of } 0.1 \text{ N iodine}$$

Due to strong reducing properties of hydriodic acid, the oxidation with iodine is a reversible reaction.

$$As_2O_3 + 2I_2 + 2H_2O \rightleftharpoons As_2O_5 + 4H^+ + 4I^-$$

The reaction proceeds to the right by removal of the hydriodic acid (HI) with sodium bicarbonate. Sodium hydroxide or sodium carbonate cannot be used to remove the HI because they react with iodine as follows :

$$6NaOH + 3I_2 \longrightarrow 5NaI + NaI + NaIO_2 + 3H_2O$$

$$3Na_2CO_3 + 3I_2 \longrightarrow 5NaI + NaIO_2 + 3CO_2$$

Procedure : An accurately weighed amount of arsenic trioxide (0.5 g) was taken in a beaker, sodium hydroxide solution (20%, 2 ml) added, and warmed to dissolve. It is cooled, transferred quantitatively to a 100 ml graduated flask and the volume adjusted. Pipette 20 ml, acidify with dilute HCl, add sodium bicarbonate to remove the excess acid, followed a further 2 g to remove the HI. Titrate with 0.1 N iodine solution to get the end point as a first permanent pale straw yellown colour.

Note : The acidification of arsenic trioxide is necessary to remove the free NaOH which would react with the iodine.

Iodine–Sodium Thiosulphate Titration : Sodium thiosulphate is oxidized to sodium tetrathionate.

$$2S_2O_3{}^{2-} \longrightarrow S_4O_6{}^{2-} + 2e^-$$
$$I_2 + 2e^- \longrightarrow 2I^-$$

Therefore, $2S_2O_3 \equiv I_2 \equiv 2e^-$

$$2 \times 248.2 \text{ g } Na_2S_2O_3.5H_2O \equiv 2000 \text{ ml N}$$
$$24.82 \text{ g } Na_2S_2O_3.5H_2O \equiv 1000 \text{ ml 0.1 N iodine}$$

Procedure : Transfer 6.025 g of accurately weighed of sodium thiosulphate to a 250 ml graduated flask, dissolve in water, adjust to volume and shake. Pipette 20 ml of 0.1 N iodine into a conical flask and titrate with the standard sodium thiosulphate solution until just colourless.

Titration of Bromine

This titration is used to determine percentage of phenol which is treated with excess of 0.1 N bromine.

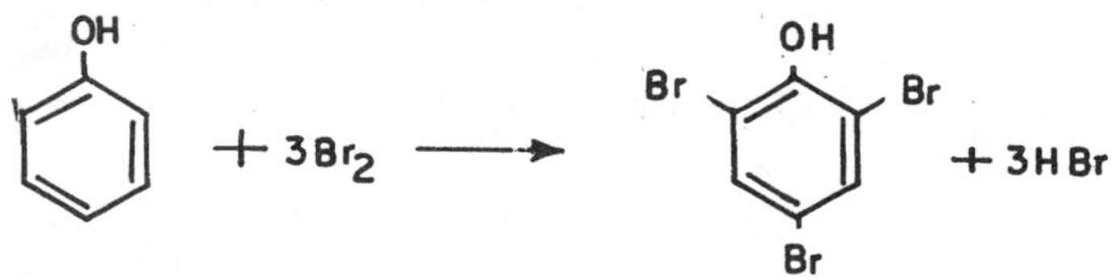

Phenol Tribromophenol

The excess of bromine not consumed in the reaction is determined by adding potassium iodide and titrating the liberated iodine with sodium thiosulphate solution.

$$Br_2 + 2I^- \longrightarrow 2Br^- + I_2$$

Therefore, $C_6H_5OH \equiv 3Br_2 \equiv 3I_2 \equiv 6e^-$

$$94.11 \text{ g of } C_6H_5OH \equiv 1 \text{ ml 0.1 N } Br_2$$

A solution of bromine is not stable. Therefore, a solution containing potassium bromide and potassium bromate is used. This solution forms bromine on acidification :

$$Br_3^- + 5Br^- + 6H^+ \longrightarrow 3Br_2 + 3H_2O$$

The amounts of potassium bromide (15 g) and potassium bromate (3 g) in water (1 litre) on acidification should produce nearly 0.1 N bromine solution. A blank titration is also carried out.

Procedure : Dissolve 2 g accurately weighed of the sample in water in 1 litre graduated flask and adjust to volume. Pipette 20 ml into a glass-stoppered bottle. Add 0.1 N bromine solution (50 ml) from a pipette and concentrated HCl(5 ml). Shake well for 30 minutes and keep for 15 minutes. Add potassium iodide (1 g), shake well, wash the stopper and titrate the liberated iodine with standard sodium thiosulphate solution. When the solution is pale yellow in colour, add chloroform (10 ml) and a few drops of starch mucilage, and titrate with vigorous shaking to a colourless end point. A blank titration is performed on the bromine-bromate solution (50 ml).

Titration in Non-aqueous Solvents

Substances with very weak acidic or very weak basic property not giving sharp end points in aqueous solution can often be titrated in non-aqueous solvents. According to the Lowry-Bronsted theory, an acid (HB) is a proton donor and a base (B) is a proton acceptor; i.e. a substance which tends to combine with a proton. When the acid dissociates, it yields a proton together with the conjugate base B of the acid.

$$HB \rightleftharpoons H^+ + B^-$$

Acid Proton Base.

A base B combines with a proton to form the conjugate acid HB of the base B. For every base, there is a conjugate acid and *vice versa.* An acid may be either an electrically neutral molecule, e.g. HCl, or a positively charged cation, e.g. $C_6H_5NH_3^+$, or a negatively charged anion, e.g. HSO_4^-. Similarly, a base may be either an electrically neutral molecule, e.g. $C_6H_5NH_2$, or an anion, e.g. Cl^-.

Acids		Bases
HCl	$\rightleftharpoons$	$H^+ + Cl^-$
HSO_4^-	$\rightleftharpoons$	$H^+ + SO_4^{2-}$
$C_6H_5NH_3^+$	$\rightleftharpoons$	$H^+ + C_6H_5NH_2$

Solvents

Aprotic Solvents : These are chemically inert organic solvents like benzene and chloroform. They have a low dielectric constant, do not react with either acids or bases and do not ionize other compounds. Picric acid forms a colourless solution in benzene which becomes yellow on adding aniline since the acid does not dissociate in benzene solution and in the presence of the base aniline, it acts as an acid.

Protophilic Solvents : These are basic in character and form solvated protons on reaction with acids.

$$\text{HB + basic solvent} \longrightarrow \text{Solvated proton} + B^-$$

A weakly basic solvent has less tendency to accept a proton than a strongly basic one. Similarly, a weak acid has less tendency to donate protons than a strong acid such as perchloric acid exhibits more strongly acidic properties than a weak acid such as acetic acid when dissolved in a weakly basic solvent. All acids tend to become typical in strength when dissolved in strongly basic solvents due to the greater affinity of strong bases for protons. This is termed as levelling effect. Strong bases are levelling solvents for acids; weak bases are differentiating solvents for acids.

Protogenic Solvents : These are acidic substances, e.g. hydrochloric acid. They exert a levelling effect on bases.

Amphiprotic Solvents : These solvents have both protophilic and protogenic properties, e.g. water, acetic acid and alcohols. They are dissociated in small amount, e.g.

$$CH_3COOH \rightleftharpoons CH_3COO^- + H^+$$

If a strong acid like perchloric acid is added in acetic acid, the acetic acid behaves as a base and combines with protons donated by the perchloric acid to form an 'Onium' ions which acts as a strongly acidic solution due to donating nature of proton to a base.

$$HClO_4 \rightleftharpoons ClO_4^- + H^+$$

$$CH_3COOH + H^+ \rightleftharpoons CH_3COOH_2^+$$

Onium ion.

When a weak base, e.g. pyridine, is dissolved in acetic acid, the acid exhibits its levelling effect and increases the basic properties of the pyridine. Therefore, it is useful to titrate a solution of a weak base in acetic acid with perchloric acid in acetic acid, and obtain a sharp end point. Titrations of these compounds in aqueous solution are not successful.

$$HClO_4 + CH_3\,COOH \rightleftharpoons CH_3COOH_2^+ + ClO_4^-$$

$$C_5H_5N + CH_3\,COOH \rightleftharpoons C_5H_5NH^+ + CH_3COO^-$$

$$CH_3COOH_2^+ + CH_3COOH^- \rightleftharpoons 2CH_3COOH$$

Therefore,

$$HClO_4 + C_5H_5N \rightleftharpoons C_5H_5NH^+ + ClO_4^-$$

Titration with Perchloric Acid : Alkali metals, alkaline earth metals, amines and pyridine are titrated with perchloric acids.

Preparation of 0.1 N Perchloric Acid : Perchloric acid (72%, 8.5 ml) is slowly added with shaking to glacial acetic acid (900 ml). Then acetic anhydride (30 ml) is added and the volume adjusted to 1 litre with glacial acetic acid. The solution is allowed to stand for 24 hours before use. The acetic anhydride reacts with water present with perchloric acid and acetic acid to give an anhydrous solution. The perchloric acid must be well diluted with acetic acid before adding acetic anhydride. Otherwise explosive acetyl perchlorate may be formed.

Standardization of 0.1 N Perchloric Acid : Alkali and alkaline earth metal salts of organic acid act as bases in acetic acid solution.

$$R\,COOM \rightleftharpoons RCOO^- + M^+$$

$$CH_3COOH_2^+ + RCOO^- \rightleftharpoons RCOOH + CH_3COOH$$

Potassium hydrogen phthalate may be used as a standardization agent for perchloric acid.

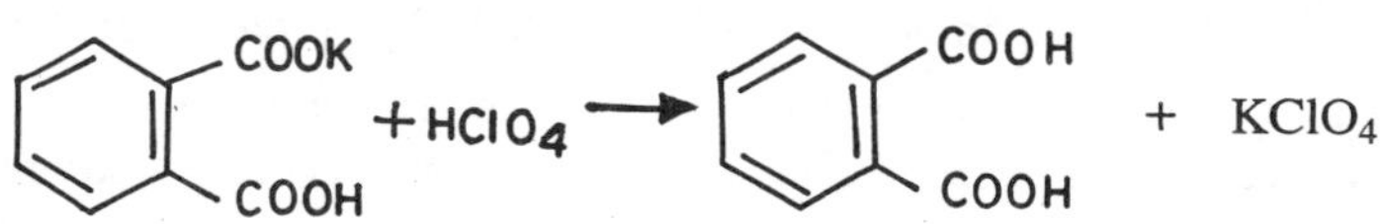

$$204.14 \text{ g of } C_8H_5O_4K \equiv HClO_4 \equiv 1000 \text{ ml N}$$

or, $$0.02041 \text{ g of } C_8H_5O_4K \equiv 1 \text{ ml } 0.1 \text{ N } HClO_4$$

Procedure : Accurately weighed quantity of potassium hydrogen phtalate (0.5 g) is poured into a 100 ml conical flask. A reflux condenser is attached with silica gel drying tube. Glacial acetic acid (25 ml) is added, warmed to dissolve salt, cooled and titrated with 0.1 N perchloric acid using 2 drops of an indicator such as 0.5% acetous crystal violet (end point blue to blue green) or 0.5 % acetous oracet blue B (end point blue to pink) or α-naphtholbenzein (0.2 % in glacial acetic acid) (end point blue to dark-green) or quinaldine red (0.1 % in methanol)(end point magenta to almost colourless).

The same indicator must be used throughout for standardization. The end point may be determined by titrating potentiometrically and plotting dE/dV against V.

Non-aqueous solvents show greater coefficients of expansion than water. A small temperature variation can resulted in significant errors unless suitable correction factors are used. Therefore, standardization and titration should be carried out at the same temperature. If there is a temperature difference, the volume of titrant may be corrected by applying the following formula :

$$V_a = V_b\,[1 + 0.001\,(t_1 - t_2)]$$

where, V_a = corrected volume of titrant

V_b = volume of titrant measured

t_1 = temperature of which titrant was standardized

t_2 = temperature at which titration was carried.

Preparation and standardization of 0.1 M Sodium Methoxide Solution

Cool down anhydrous methanol (150 ml) in ice-cold water and add freshly cut sodium metal (about 2.5 g) in portions. When the metal has dissolved, add sufficient amount of toluene, previously dried over sodium wire, to produce 1000 ml. Standardize the solution in the following manner immediately before use.

Dissolve accurately weighed benzoic acid (0.4 g) in dimethylformamide (80 ml), add thymolphthalein solution (0.15 ml) and titrate with sodium methoxide solution to a blue end point.

Factor : Each ml of 0.1 M sodium methoxide is equivalent to 0.01221 g of benzoic acid.

Note : Protect the solution from atmospheric carbon dioxide throughout the titration.

Sodium Nitrite Titrations

When aromatic primary amines are reacted with sodium nitrite in acid solution at low temperature (0–4°C), diazonium salts are formed.

$$C_6H_5NH_2 + NaNO_2 + HCl \xrightarrow{0\text{–}4^\circ C} \underset{\text{Diazonium salt}}{C_6H_5N_2Cl} + NaCl + 2H_2O$$

Under controlled conditions the reaction is quantitative and used for determination of free aromatic amines as in sulphanilamide and other sulpha drugs. The presence of a small excess of nitrous acid indicates the end point which is detected using starch — iodide paper as an external indicator.

$$KI + HCl \longrightarrow HI + KCl$$

$$2HI + 2HNO_2 \longrightarrow I_2 + 2NO + 2H_2O$$

The liberated iodine reacts with starch to form a blue colour.

The end point may also be detected electrometrically.

Determination of Sodium Aminosalicylate

Treatment of sodium aminosalicylate ($C_7H_6NNaO_3$) with sodium nitrite forms a diazonium salt.

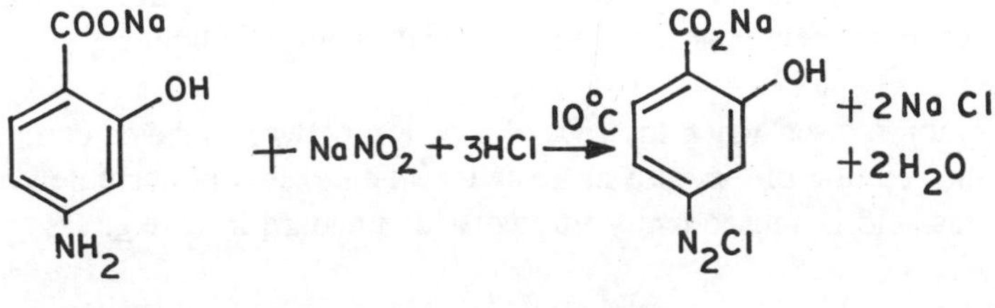

$$175.2 \text{ g of } C_7H_6NNaO_3 \equiv NaNO_2 \equiv 1000 \text{ ml M}$$

or $$0.01752 \text{ g of } C_7H_6NNaO_3 \equiv 1 \text{ ml } 0.1 \text{ M } NaNO_2$$

Procedure : Weigh accurately about 0.25 g and dissolve in glacial acetic acid (50 ml), warm gently, if necessary. Add cold water (175 ml) and cool below 10°, add hydrochloric acid (10 ml) and slowly titrate with 0.1 M sodium nitrite at a temperature below 10° until a drop of the solution immediately gives a blue colour when drawn quickly by means of a fine rod across the surface of a starch iodide paper. The titration is complete when the end point is reproducable after the titrated solution has been allowed to stand for 6 minutes.

The end point may be determined by electrometric method.

3

Volumetric Analysis

It is a quite accurate method of quantitative analysis. The quantity of a substance in a solution is determined by accurately measuring the volume of the reacting solution.

Volumetric analysis may be classified into various categories based on type of reactions involved, e.g.:

(1) Neutralization titration or acidimetry and alkalimetry

(2) Precipitation titration

(3) Oxidation-Reduction titration

(4) Complexometric titration

(5) Non-aqueous titration

(6) Diazotization titration

NEUTRALIZATION TITRATION

It involves the neutralization of an acid with a base or vice versa. End point is determined by means of an indicator.

Acidimetry Titration

It is a direct or residual volumetric analysis of a base with a standard acid.

Direct titration is performed by introducing a standard acid solution gradually from a burette into a solution of base being assayed till the end point is obtained, e.g. assay of sodium bicarbonate.

Residual titration is used when the rate of reaction between a basic compound with an acid is slow. In this, the solution of the base in treated with an excess of accurately measured standard acid and the excess acid is subsequently titrated with standard base, e.g. assay of zinc oxide.

Direct Titration

Assay of Sodium Bicarbonate

Sodium bicarbonate I.P. contains not less than 99% and not more than the equivalent of 100.5% of $NaHCO_3$ calculated with reference of the dried substance.

Procedure: Accurately weigh about 1 g of sodium bicarbonate and dissolve in water (20 ml). Titrate the solution with 0.5 N sulphuric acid solution by using methyl orange as an indicator till yellow colour is changed into pink colour.

$$2NaHCO_3 + H_2SO_4 \longrightarrow Na_2SO_4 + 2H_2O + 2CO_2$$

Methyl orange is used as the indicator because phenolphthalein is affected by carbonic acid liberated in the reaction which may cause a change of colour before completion of the reaction.

Factor : 1 ml of 0.5 N H_2SO_4 is equivalent to 0.042 g of $NaHCO_3$.

Assay of Sodium Carbonate

Sodium carbonate contains not less than 99% and not more than the equivalent of 105% of $Na_2CO_3.10H_2O$.

Aqueous solution of sodium carbonate is alkaline in nature. It is assayed by titrating with a standard acid using bromophenol blue as an indicator. At the end point, acidic pH is obtained due to formation of carbonic acid from carbon dioxide.

$$Na_2CO_3 + H_2SO_4 \longrightarrow Na_2SO_4 + H_2O + CO_2$$

Hence, bromophenol blue is a choice of indicator as it shows colour change in acidic range. The pH range of bromophenol blue is 2.8 to 4.6.

Procedure : Weigh accurately sodium carbonate (2 g), dissolve in water (20 ml) and titrate with 0.5 N sulphuric acid solution by using bromophenol as an indicator till yellow colour is obtained.

Factor : Each ml of 0.5 N H_2SO_4 is equivalent to 0.0715 g of Na_2CO_3.

Assay of Borax, $Na_2B_4O_7$, $10H_2O$

Borax was an official in I.P. 1966. It contains not less than 99% and not more than the equivalent of 103% of $Na_2B_4O_7$.

Procedure : Weigh accurately about 3 g, dissolve in water (75 ml) and titrate with 0.5 N hydrochloric acid using solution of methyl red as indicator.

On titration with hydrochloric acid, boric acid is formed.

$$2HCl + Na_2B_4O_7 + 5H_2O \longrightarrow 2NaCl + 4H_3BO_3.$$

The colour changes when all the boric acid has been set free. Boric acid has a very low ionisation and has no effect on indicators. Methyl red changes its colour in the range 4.2—6.3 and hence is not affected by free boric acid.

Each ml of 0.5 N hydrochloric acid = 0.09536 g of $Na_2B_4O_7.10H_2O$.

Residual Titration

Assay of Strong Ammonia Solution :

Strong ammonia solution contains not less then 24.5% w/w and not more than 25.5% w/w of NH_3.

The ammonia solution is assayed by residual or back titration due to its volatile nature, otherwise some quantity may lost during direct titration with a standard acid.

Ammonia solution is treated with an accurately measured standard acid and the standard acid is back titrated with a standard alkali by using methyl red as an indicator.

$$2NH_3 + H_2SO_4 \longrightarrow (NH_4)_2SO_4.$$

Procedure : Weigh accurately ammonia solution (3 g) in a flask containing 1 N sulphuric acid (50 ml) and titrate the excess of acid with 1 N sodium hydroxide solution by using methyl red as an indicator till yellow colour is changed into red colour.

Factor : Each ml of 1 N H_2SO_4 is equivalent to 0.01703 g of NH_3.

Assay of Zinc Oxide : Zinc oxide contains not less than 99% and not more than the equivalent of 100.5% of ZnO, calculated with reference to the ignited substance.

Accurately weighed amounts of zinc oxide (1.5 g) and ammonium chloride (2.5 g) are dissolved in 1N sulphuric acid solution (50 ml) with the aid of gentle heating. Titrate the solution with 1N sodium hydroxide solution till yellow colour is obtained.

$$ZnO + H_2SO_4 \longrightarrow ZnSO_4 + H_2O.$$

It is back titrated due to slow reaction between zinc oxide and sulphuric acid. Ammonium chloride is added to prevent the precipitation of zinc hydroxide both during the titration and also at the end point. The precipitation of zinc hydroxide would give poor end point.

Factor : Each ml of 1N H_2SO_4 is equivalent to 0.04068 g of ZnO.

Alkalimetry Titration

It is an estimation of acid/acidic drugs by titration with standard alkali. It also includes direct titration and residual/back titration methods as in acidimetry.

Direct Titration

Assay of Boric Acid (H_3BO_3)

Boric acid I.P. contains not less than 99.5% and not more than the equivalent of 100.5% of H_3BO_3 calculated with reference to the dried substance.

Procedure: Accurately weigh boric acid (2 g) and dissolve in a mixture of water (50 ml) and glycerin (100 ml), previously neutralized to phenolphthalein indicator. Titrate the solution with 1 N sodium hydroxide solution by using phenolphthalein as indicator till pink colour is obtained.

Boric acid is a weak acid, hence it cannot be titrated accurately with standard alkali. It can be titrated directly after dissolving in a solution of glycerin or polyhydroxy compound, e.g. manitol, in water. In the above method, boric acid reacts with glycerin to form glyceroboric acid which is a strong monobasic acid.

Glycerin is slightly acidic in nature. Therefore, it is neutralized with dilute alkali solution, using phenolphthalein indicator.

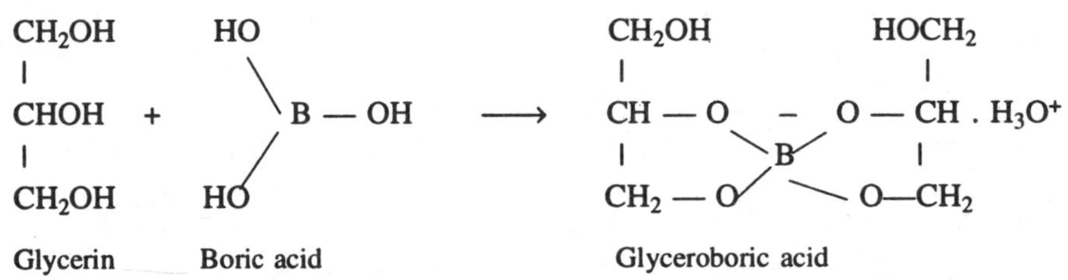

Factor : Each ml of 1 N NaOH is equivalent to 0.06183 g of H_3BO_3

Assay of Ammonium Chloride : Ammonium chloride contains not less than 99.5% of NH_4Cl calculated with reference to the dried substances.

Procedure : Weigh accurately ammonium chloride (about 0.1 g), dissolve in water (20 ml) and add formaldehyde solution (5 ml), previously neutralized to phenolphthalein indicator. After two minutes, titrate slowly with 0.1 N sodium hydroxide solution by using phenolphthalein indicator till pink colour is obtained.

The above method is official in I.P. 1985 while precipitation method is recommended in I.P. 1966. In this method, ammonium chloride is treated with formaldehyde solution to liberate equivalent amount of hydrochloric acid which is titrated with 0.1 N sodium hydroxide solution.

$$HCl + NaOH \longrightarrow NaCl + H_2O$$

Factor : 1000 ml of 0.1 N NaOH is equivalent to 0.005349 g of NH_4Cl.

Residual Titration

In this, acid is treated with excess of accurately measured base which is then titrated with a standard acid.

Assay of Aspirin

It contains not less than 99.5% and not more than the equivalent of 100.5% of aspirin calculated with reference to the dried substance.

Procedure : Weigh accurately aspirin (1.5 g), add 0.5 N sodium hydroxide solution (50 ml) and boil for 10 minutes. Cool the solution and titrate the excess of alkali with 0.5 N sulphuric acid solution using phenol red indicator. Perform a blank titration in the same way.

On boiling with standard sodium hydroxide solution, aspirin is hydrolyzed into salicylic acid and acetic acid. The liberated acid reacts with sodium hydroxide to form sodium salt. At the end point, a slight excess of the base reacts with the indicator to produce colour change.

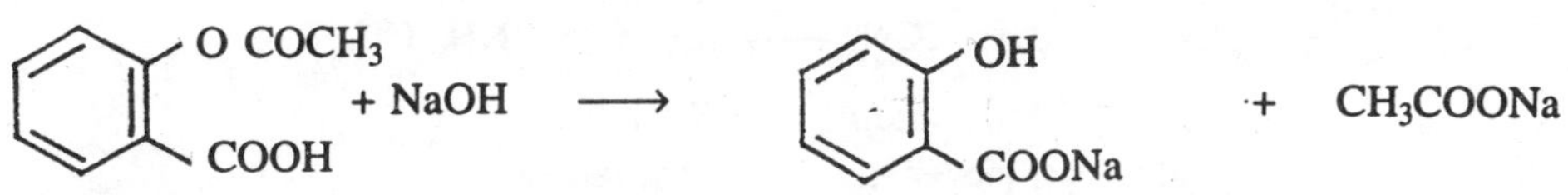

Aspirin Sodium Salicylate

Factor : Each ml of 0.5 N NaOH is equivalent to 0.04504 g of $C_9 H_8 O_4$.

PRECIPITATION TITRATIONS

It involves the formation of insoluble substances or precipitates. End point is detected by observing the completion of precipitation or by the use of internal indicator. It is classified into :

(1) Direct titration method and

(2) Residual or Indirect titration method

1. Direct Titration Method

The substance in solution is directly titrated with a titrant (precipitant) and completion of precipitation is detected by the use of an internal indicator.

Assay of Sodium Chloride (NaCl) : It contains not less than 99.5 % and not more than the equivalent of 100.5% of sodium chloride calculated with reference to the dried substance.

Procedure : Accurately weigh sodium chloride (about 0.25 g), dissolve in water (50 ml) and titrate with 0.1N silver nitrate using an potassium chromate as an indicator.

Sodium chloride is precipitated as silver chloride by adding silver nitrate solution.

$$NaCl + AgNO_3 \longrightarrow AgCl\downarrow + NaNO_3$$

White precipitate

When the precipitate formation is completed, a drop of silver nitrate reacts with the indicator, potassium chromate, to form a red precipitate of silver chromate.

$$2AgNO_3 + K_2CrO_4 \longrightarrow \underset{\text{Silver chromate}}{Ag_2CrO_4} + 2KNO_3$$

This method is also called Mohr's method and is applicable if the solution to be titrated is neutral. In acid solution, potassium chromate cannot be used as the indicator due to solubility of silver chromate in acids.

Factor : 1 ml of 0.1 N $AgNO_3$ is equivalent to 0.005854 g of NaCl.

2. Residual Titrations Method

This method is also called Volhard's method and is applicable for acidic salts also. In this excess of standard silver nitrate is added to a solution of halide acidified with nitric acid. The unreacted silver nitrate is titrated with standard ammonium thiocyanate solution using ferric ammonium sulphate as an indicator.

At the end point, a permanent red colour is developed due to formation of ferric ferrithiocyanate.

Bromides and iodides can be estimated by Volhard's method without any modification but in the case of chloride, nitrobenzene is added or precipitate of silver chloride is filtered off. Nitrobenzene forms a protective layer on the precipitate of silver chloride (coagulation). The precipitate of silver chloride, if not removed or coagulated, reacts slowly with ammonium thiocyanate (reading will be high.)

$$\underset{\text{Silver chloride}}{AgCl} + \underset{\text{Ammonium thiocyanate}}{NH_4SCN} \longrightarrow \underset{\text{Silver thiocyanate}}{AgSCN} + NH_4Cl$$

Assay of Sodium Chloride (I.P. 1985 official method) :

Procedure : Weigh accurately sodium chloride (0.2 g), dissolve in distilled water (50 ml), and then add 0.1 N silver nitrate solution (50 ml), nitric acid (3 ml) and nitrobenzene (5 ml). Shake the solution, add ferric ammonium sulphate indicator and titrate with 0.1 N ammonium thiocyanate solution till the colour becomes reddish yellow.

Sodium chloride is precipitated as silver chloride by addition of excess of silver nitrate solution. The precipitate of silver chloride is coagulated by nitrobenzene.

$$NaCl + AgNO_3 \longrightarrow AgCl + NaNO_3$$

The excess of silver nitrate reacts with ammonium thiocyanate on titration. When whole amount is consumed, a drop of ammonium thiocyanate reacts with ferric ammonium sulphate indicator to give reddish yellow colour.

$$AgNO_3 + NH_4SCN \longrightarrow AgSCN + NH_4NO_3$$

$$NH_4SCN + FeNH_4(SO_4)_2 \longrightarrow \underset{\text{Ferric thiocyanate (red colour)}}{Fe(SCN)_3} + 2(NH_4)_2SO_4$$

Factor : Each ml of 0.1 N $AgNO_3$ solution is equivalent to 0.0005845 g of NaCl.

Assay of Ammonium Chloride by Volhard's Method

Procedure (Official in I.P. 1966) : official in I.P. 1966. Accurately weigh ammonium chloride (0.2 g) dissolve in distilled water (40 ml), add nitric acid (3 ml), nitrobenzene (5 ml) and 0.1 N $AgNO_3$ solution (50 ml), shake vigorously for one minute and titrate with 0.1 N ammonium thiocyanate using ferric ammonium sulphate as the indicator.

Now the above method is replaced by acid-base titration in I.P. 1985 (refer Acidimetry).

Ammonium chloride is precipitated by adding excess of silver nitrate. The unreacted silver nitrate is estimated by titration with standard ammonium thiocyanate solution. At the end point, a drop of NH_4SCN reacts with ferric ammonium sulphate indicator to give red colour.

$$NH_4Cl + AgNO_3 \longrightarrow AgNO_3 + NH_4NO_3$$

$$FeNH_4(SO_4)_2 + NH_4SCN \longrightarrow Fe(SCN)_3 + 2(NH_4)_2SO_4$$

Ferric thiocyanate (red colour)

Factor : Each ml of 0.1 N $AgNO_3$ solution is equivalent to 0.005349 g of NH_4Cl.

OXIDATION-REDUCTION TITRATIONS

Oxidation and reduction occur simultaneously in oxidation-reduction reaction. The reactant which losses electron is the reducing agent and can be identified as the reactant containing a constituent atom or atoms converted to higher state of oxidation.

$$Fe^{++} \longrightarrow Fe^{3+} + e^- \text{ (loss of electron)}$$

Ferrous (ion) Ferric (ion)

The electrons lost by the reducing agent are gained by the oxidizing agent, the reactant containing a constituent atom or atoms which are converted to a lower state of oxidation. e.g.

$$Fe^{3+} + e^- \longrightarrow Fe^{++} \text{ (gain of electron)}$$

Ferric Ferrous

A combination of oxidizing and reducing agents results in oxidation-reduction reaction which forms the basis for quantitative measurement of one of the reactants. A standard solution of oxidizing agent can be used for estimation of reducing agent, e.g. potassium permanganate is an oxidizing agent and can be used in quantitative estimation of the reducing agent, ferrous sulphate. Similarly sodium thiosulphate, a reducing agent, can be used for iodine which is an oxidizing agent. Oxidation-reduction methods can be classified on the basis of oxidizing agents.

Permanganate Methods : It involves the use of potassium permanganate for estimation of number of reducing substances, e.g. ferrous sulphate.

Potassium permanganate also serves as a self indicator. As a very slight excess of permanganate, it gives a distinct pink colour to the solution due to manganese ion.

Assay of Ferrous Sulphate

Ferrous sulphate contains not less than 98% and not more than equivalent of 105% of $FeSO_4.7H_2O$.

Procedure : Weigh accurately ferrous sulphate (1 g), dissolve in dilute sulphuric acid (20 ml) and titrate with 0.1 N $KMnO_4$ solution till faint pink colour persists for about 30 seconds upon shaking the flask.

This method was official in I.P. 1966. Ferrous sulphate is oxidized by potassium permanganate into ferric sulphate. When whole ferrous sulphate is consumed, a drop of potassium permanganate solution gives pink colour at the end point.

$$10\ FeSO_4 + 2KMnO_4 \longrightarrow 5\ Fe_2(SO_4)_3 + 2MnSO_4 + K_2\ SO_4 + 8H_2O$$

Factor : Each ml of 0.1 N $KMnO_4$ solution is equivalent to 0.0278 g of $FeSO_4 \cdot 7H_2O$.

Assay of Sodium Nitrite

Procedure : Dissolve accurately weighed sodium nitrite (1 g) in water to make 100 ml solution in volumetric flask. Add this solution (10 ml) into a mixture of 0.1 N potassium permanganate solution (50 ml), sulfuric acid (5 ml) and water (100 ml).

Precaution : Immerse the tip of pipette beneath the surface of potassium permanganate solution while adding the sodium nitrite solution.

Warm the mixture to 40°, add 0.1 N oxalic acid (25 ml). Heat the mixture to 60° on a water bath and titrate with 0.1 N potassium permanganate solution till pink colour persists for 30 seconds after shaking.

It is a back titration. Sodium nitrite is oxidized with potassium permanganate into sodium nitrate.

$$10\ NaNO_2 + 4KMnO_4 + 11H_2SO_4 \longrightarrow 10\ HNO_3 + 4MnSO_4 + 2K_2SO_4 + 5Na_2SO_4 + 6H_2O$$

Sodium nitrite yields nitrous acid in the presence of sulphuric acid which is volatile; it would be lost if no precaution is taken while adding the sodium nitrite solution by keeping the tip of pipette beneath the surface of the acidified potassium permanganate solution.

Instead of titrating excess of potassium permanganate solution with standard oxalic acid to disappearance of pink colour, the excess of potassium permanganate is reduced by adding an excess amount of oxalic acid and titrating the excess of oxalic acid with parmanganate to the appearance of pink colour. This sequence is followed because it is easy to detect the appearance of pink colour.

Factor : Each ml 0.1 N $KMnO_4$ is equivalent to 0.00345 g of $NaNO_2$.

Assay of Hydrogen Peroxide

It is an aqueous solution containing hydrogen peroxide, not less than 5% w/v and not more than 7.0% w/v of H_2O_2 corresponding to 20 volume strength . It has not more than 0.025% w/v of suitable stabilising agent. Twenty volume strength means that it gives 20 times its volume of oxygen on complete decomposition by heat.

Procedure : Dilute hydrogen peroxide (10 to 25 ml) with water, add 5 N sulphuric acid solution (5 ml) and titrate with 0.1 N potassium permanganate solution to a permanent pink end point.

Hydrogen peroxide has both oxidizing and reducing properties, but if titrated against an acidified potassium permanganate solution (stronger oxidizing agent), it acts as a reducing agent. When hydrogen peroxide is reacted with potassium permanganate, it is oxidized into oxygen. High concentration of the acid is used to prevent the formation of manganese dioxide which may cause decomposition of hydrogen peroxide.

$$5H_2O_2 + 2KMnO_4 + 3H_2SO_4 \longrightarrow 5O_2\uparrow + 2MnSO_4 + K_2SO_4 + 8H_2O$$

Factor : Each ml of 0.1 N $KMnO_4$ solution is equivalent to 0.01701 g of H_2O_2.

IODIMETRIC AND IODOMETRIC METHODS

It involves the use of iodine as a mild oxidizing agent. It can be used for estimation of reducing agents, e.g. sodium thiosulphate. Such direct method is called 'Iodimetry'. In the indirect method, known as Iodometry, the oxidizing agent is reduced with excess of potassium iodide to liberate an equivalent amount of iodine which can be estimated by titrating with standard sodium thiosulphate. Iodometry is used for assays of copper sulphate, available chlorine, etc.

Assay of Iodine

Iodine contains not less than 99.5% and not more than equivalent of 100.5% of I.

Procedure : Weigh accurately iodine (0.5 g) and dissolve in a solution of potassium iodide (1 g) in H_2O (5 ml).. Dilute it with water to 25 ml, acidify with acetic acid (1 ml) and titrate with 0.1 N sodium thiosulphate till light yellow colour is obtained. At this stage, add starch mucilage and the titration is continued till blue colour disappears.

It is iodimetric method, official in I.P. 1985. Iodine is directly estimated by titration with the reducing agent, sodium thiosulphate ($Na_2S_2O_3$) .

$$I_2 + \underset{\text{Sodium thiosulphate}}{Na_2S_2O_3} \longrightarrow \underset{\text{Sodium tetrathionate}}{Na_2S_4O_6} + 2NaI$$

Starch is added toward the end of titration, when most of iodine is reacted with sodium thiosulphate as starch mucilage forms stable complex with excess of iodine.

Factor : Each ml of 0.1 N $Na_2S_2O_3$ is equivalent to 0.01269 g of I.

Aqueous Iodine Solution

Synonym : Lugol's solution

It contains 5% w/v of iodine (limits 4.9 to 5.1%) and 10% w/v of potassium iodide (limits 9.8 to 10.2)

Procedure : Estimation is carried for both iodine and potassium iodide. Aqueous iodine solution (25 ml) is diluted to 100 ml with water.

For Iodine : To the above solution (20 ml), water (10 ml) is added and titrated with 0.1 N sodium thiosulphate by using starch mucilage as indicator till blue colour disappears.

Each ml of 0.1 N $Na_2S_2O_3$ is equivalent to 0.012698 of I.

For Potassium Iodide : To the above diluted solution (10 ml), water (20 ml) and conc. HCl (40 ml) are added and them titrated wih 0.05 M potassium iodate (KIO_3) solution, with vigorous shaking until dark blue solution becomes only light brown in colour. Chloroform (5 ml) is added and the titration continued until chloroform becomes colourless and supernatent liquid is clear yellow. From the number of ml of 0.05 M potassium iodate solution required, substract one quarter of the number of ml of 0.1 N sodium thiosulphate required in the assay for iodine.

Each ml of 0.05 M KIO_3 solution is equivalent to 0.01668 of KI.

Iodides are quantitatively oxidized by iodate to iodine which reacts with more iodate in presence of strong hydrochloric acid to form iodine monochloride (ICl).

$$5KI + KIO_3 + 6HCl \longrightarrow 3I_2 + 6KCl + 3H_2O \quad .... (1)$$

$$2I_2 + KIO_3 + 6HCl \longrightarrow KCl + 5ICl + 3H_2O \quad .... (2)$$

Starch mucilage cannot be used in this titration due to high concentration of hydrochloric acid (hydrolysis of starch occurs). Iodine monochloride is stable in high concentration of the acid. The end point is detected by disappearance of violet colour of iodine in chloroform.

In the above equation (2), one mole of KIO_3 reacts with 2 moles of iodine (four atoms of iodine atoms). Hence M/20 KIO_3 is equivalent to M/5 iodine and a litre of M/5 iodine is equivalent to 1000 ml of M/5 sodium thiosulphate or 2000 ml of M/10 sodium thiosulphate. If one quater volume of N/10 sodium thiosulphate used for titrating iodine is substracted from the volume of M/20 KIO_3 used; the difference is a measure of potassium iodide in the solution.

Assay of Copper Sulphate

It contains not less than 98.5% and not more than the equivalent of 101% of $CuSO_4.5H_2O$.

Procedure : Weigh accurately copper sulphate (1 g), dissolve in water (50 ml), add potassium iodide (3 g) and acetic acid (5 ml) and titrate the liberated iodine with 0.1 N sodium thiosulphate till light yellow colour is obtained. At this stage starch mucilage and potassium thiocyanate (2 g) are added and the titration is continued until blue colour disappears.

Copper sulphate is assayed by iodometric method. Reducing agent, KI, is added in presence of acetic acid to form cupric iodide. Acetic acid is added to form a weakly acidic solution.

Cupric iodide is unstable and decomposes into cuprous iodide and iodine. The liberated iodine is titrated with sodium thiosulphate till the solution becomes yellow. Most of the liberated iodine is reacted with sodium thiosulphate, little amount is left (indicated by yellow colour).

Starch mucilage is added towards the end because it forms stable complex with excess of iodine.

$$2CuSO_4 + 4KI \longrightarrow 2CuI_2 + 2K_2SO_4$$

$$\underset{\text{Cupric iodide}}{2CuI_2} \rightleftharpoons \underset{\text{Cuprous iodide}}{Cu_2I_2} + I_2$$

$$I_2 + 2Na_2S_4O_6 \longrightarrow 2Na_2S_4O_6 + 2NaI$$

The decomposition of cupric iodide into cuprous iodide and iodine is reversible, hence to make quantitative, potassium thiocyanate is added which reacts with the reaction product, cuprous iodide, to form cuprous thiocyanate. Potassium thiocyanate is added toward the end of the titration to avoid errors due to absorption of iodine by cuprous thiocyanate.

$$CuI_2 + KCNS \longrightarrow \underset{\text{Cuprous thiocyanate}}{CuCNS} + 2KI$$

Factor : Each ml of 0.1 N $Na_2S_2O_3$ is equivalent to 0.02497 g of $CuSO_4.5H_2O$.

Assay of Chlorinated Lime (Synonyms : Bleaching Powder)

It contains not less than 30 % w/w of available chlorine.

Procedure : Triturate accurately weighed bleaching powder (4 g) with little quantity of water in a mortar and transfer to a 2 litre flask. Add sufficient water to make 1000 ml. Take this suspension 100 ml), add potassium iodide (3 g) dissolved in water (100 ml), acidify with acetic acid (5 ml) and titrate the liberated iodine with 0.1 N sodium thiosulphate, using starch mucilage as indicator.

It is a iodometric method, official in I.P. 1966. On acidification with acetic acid, chlorine is liberated which displaces an equivalent amount of iodine from potassium iodide. The liberated iodine is measured by titration with sodium thiosulphate solution. Starch mucilage is added towards the end of titration. Disappearance of blue colour is an indication of the end point.

$$CaCl(OCl) + 2CH_3COOH \longrightarrow Ca(CH_3COO)_2 + HCl + HOCl$$

$$HCl + HOCl \longrightarrow 2KCl + I_2$$

(Hypochlorus acid)

$$I_2 + 2Na_2S_2O_3 \longrightarrow Na_2S_4O_6 + 2NaCl$$

Factor : Each ml of 0.1 N $Na_2S_2O_3$ is equivalent to 0.003455 g of available chlorine.

Ceric Sulphate Titration Method

Solution of ceric sulphate in dilute sulphuric acid is a strong oxidizing agent and has many advantages over potassium permanganate, e.g.

(i) The solution is stable on boiling.

(ii) The cerous ion is colourless and does not cause any hindrance in detecting end point.

(iii) Ceric (Ce^{3+}) on reduction gives Ce^{4+} (Cerum). There is no intermediate product while permanganate can be reduced to any of several oxidation states.

(iv) Ferrous phenanthroline ion (ferrous) is a satisfactory indicator in the titration with ceric sulphate.

Assay of Ferrous Sulphate by Ceric Sulphate Titration Method

Procedure : Weigh accurately ferrous sulphate (1 g), dissolve in a mixture of water (30 ml) and dilute sulphuric acid (20 ml) and titrate with 0.1N ceric ammonium sulphate using O-phenanthroline- ferrous complex (ferroin) as an indicator.

This method is official in I.P. 1985 (permanganate method is official in I.P. 1966). Ferrous sulphate is oxidized into ferric sulphate in acidified solution.

$$2FeSO_4 + Ce(SO_4)_2 \longrightarrow Fe_2(SO_4)_3 + Ce_2\,(SO_4)_3$$

Ceric sulphate Cerum sulphate

At the end point, whole ferrous sulphate is reacted with ceric sulphate and then with indicator O-phenanthroline-ferrous complex (ferroin) (red colour) which is oxidized into O-phenthroline-ferric complex (blue colour).

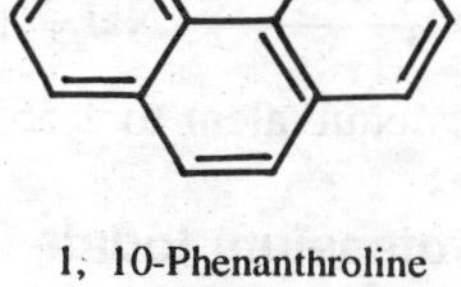

1, 10-Phenanthroline

$$C_{12}H_8N_2 \quad + \quad Fe^{++} \longrightarrow [Fe(C_{12}H_8N_2)_3]^{2+} \rightleftharpoons [Fe(C_{12}H_8N_2)_3\,]^{3+} + e^-$$

o-Phenanthroline (Colourless) — o-Phenanthroline ferrous complex (Red) — o-Phanthroline-ferric complex (Blue)

Factor : Each ml of 0.1 N ceric ammonium sulphate in equivalent to 0.002788 g of $FeSO_4.7H_2O$.

Oxidation Reduction Method with 0.1 N Bromine : Bromine is an oxidizing agent used for assay of a number of compounds, e.g. aniline, phenol, etc. as it reacts quantitatively and forms insoluble substitution products, tribromoaniline and tribromophenol, respectively. Standard bromine solution does not contain bromine as such but an equivalent amount of potassium bromide and potassium bromate ($KBrO_3$) which on acidification liberates bromine.

$$5KBr + KBrO_3 + 6HCl \longrightarrow 6KCl + 3Br_2 + 3H_2O$$

Assay of Phenol

Phenol contains not less than 98% and not more than equivalent of 100.5% of C_6H_6O calculated with reference to the anhydrous substance.

Procedure : Weigh accurately phenol (0.5 g) and dissolve in sufficient amount of water to produce 500 ml. Mix this solution (25 ml) with 0.1 N potassium bromate (25 ml) in 250 ml glass stoppered flask and add potassium bromide (1 g) and dilute hydrochloric acid (10 ml). Insert the stopper, previously moistened with a few drops of 10% w/v solution of potassium iodide and keep it in dark for 20 minute with frequent shaking. Add 10% w/v solution of potassium iodide (10 ml) and keep it in the dark for further 5 minutes with frequent shaking. Wash the stopper and neck of flask with water, add chloroform (10 ml) and titrate the liberated iodine with 0.1N sodium thiosulphate solution using starch mucilage as an indicator. Perform a blank titration in the same way.

When the hydrochloric acid is added, bromine is liberated, which reacts with phenol to form white crystalline precipitate of tribromophenol and hydrobromic acid.

$$5KBr + KBrO_3 + 6HCl \longrightarrow 6\ KCl + 3Br_2 + 3H_2O$$

$$\underset{\text{Phenol}}{C_6H_5OH} + 3Br_2 \longrightarrow \underset{\text{Tribromophenol}}{C_6H_2Br_3OH} + 3HBr$$

The flask should be stoppered to prevent the escape of the volatile bromine. Sufficient time should be given to complete oxidation of phenol to tribromophenol.

Potassium iodide liberates an equivalent amount of iodine when reacted with unreacted bromine.

$$2KI + Br_2 \longrightarrow 2KBr + I_2$$

Chloroform is added to dissolve the precipitated tribromophenol otherwise it would interfere in the detection of end point.

The liberated free iodine reacts with sodium thiosulphate. At the end point blue colour disappears as the whole of iodine is consumed with sodium thiosulphate.

$$I_2 + 2Na_2\ S_2\ O_3 \longrightarrow 2NaI + Na_2S_4O_6$$

Factor : Each ml of 0.1 N bromine is equivalent to 1.569 g of phenol.

Oxidation-Reduction Method with Potassium Iodate

In this method, potassium iodate is used as oxidizing agent. It involves the formation of iodine monochloride. A number of reducing agents, e.g. potassium iodide, can be estimated by this method.

Assay of Potassium Iodide

Potassium iodide contains not less than 99% of KI calculated with reference to the dried substance.

Procedure : Weigh accurately potassium iodide (0.5 g), dissolve in water (10 ml) and add hydrochloric acid (25 ml) and chloroform (5 ml). Titrate it with 0.05 M potassium iodate until purple colour disappears from the chloroform layer.

Potassium iodate oxidizes quantitatively iodides into iodine.

$$5KI + KIO_3 + 6HCl \longrightarrow 3I_2 + 6KCl + 3H_2O$$

The liberated iodine reacts with excess of iodate in the presence of strong hydrochloric acid to form iodine monochloride (ICl).

$$2I_2 + KIO_3 + 6HCl \longrightarrow KCl + 5ICl + 3H_2O$$

In the titration, starch mucilage can not be used as an indicator due to presence of strong hydrochloric acid which may be hydrolyzed, hence, chloroform is used. Iodine is more soluble in chloroform. The solution becomes colourless when whole iodine reacts with iodate.

COMPLEXOMETRIC TITRATIONS

Earlier aluminium and magnesium salts were assayed by a time consuming gravimetric method but with the introduction of chelate forming agents, mainly disodium salt of ethylenediamine-tetra-acetic acid, a new volumetric method is developed. It involves the formation of complex of which stability depends on pH of the solution. This method is called complexometric titration.

Assay of Calcium Carbonate

Calcium carbonate contains not less than 98% and not more than the equivalent of 100.5% of $CaCO_3$ calculated with reference to the dried substance.

Procedure : Weigh accurately of calcium carbonate (0.1 g) and dissolve in dilute hydrochloric acid (3 ml) in water (10 ml). Boil for 10 minutes, cool, dilute to 50 ml with water. Titrate with 0.05 M disodium ethylenediamine tetra-acetate (to within a few ml of expected end point), then add sodium hydroxide (8 ml) and calcon mixture (0.1 g) and continue the titration until the colour of the solution changes from pink to full blue colour.

Calcium carbonate forms complex with 0.05 M disodium ethylenediamine tetra-acetate.

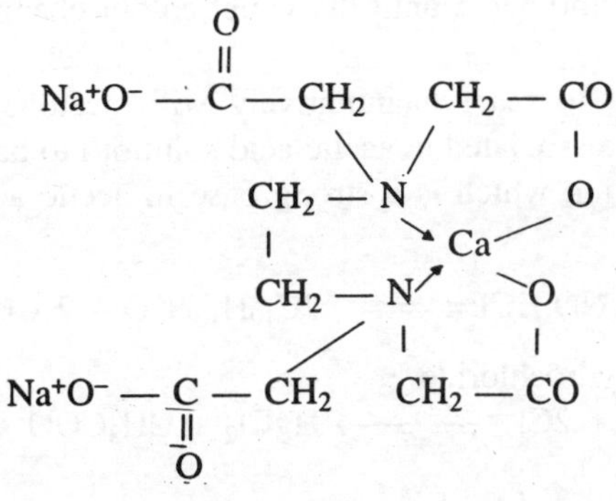

Calcium complex.

Calcon mixture is added as an indicator. It is pink in colour in the presence of calcium salt (calcium-indicator complex) but blue in colour in the absence of calcium carbonate, hence at the end point blue colour is obtained. Indicator is added towards the end of titration. Sodium hydroxide is added to maintain the alkaline pH.

Factor : Each ml of 0.05 M disodium ethylenediamine tetra-acetate is equivalent to 0.0050048 g of $CaCO_3$.

Assay of Magnesium Sulphate

Magnesium sulphate contains not less than 99% and not more than equivalent of 100% of $MgSO_4$, calculated with reference to ignited substance.

Procedure : Weigh accurately the substance (0.3 g) and dissolve in water (50 ml). Add strong ammonia- ammonium chloride solution (10 ml) and titrate with 0.05 M disodium ethylenediamine tetra-acetate using mordant black 11 mixture (0.1 g) as an indicator until pink colour is changed into blue.

Magnesium forms complex with 0.05 M disodium ethylenediamine tetra-acetate at pH 10 maintained by adding ammonia buffer. Mordant black 11 mixture is used as an indicator. The colour change at the end point is from pink to blue.

Factor : Each ml of 0.05 M disodium ethylenediamine tetra-acetate is equivalent to 0.00602 g of $MgSO_4$.

NON-AQUEOUS TITRATION

This method is used when the substance is insoluble in water or it is weak acid or weak base in comparison to water. It is again classified into

(i) Acidimetry

(ii) Alkalimetry

Acidimetry

The estimation of weak base can be performed in glacial acetic acid using perchloric acid as the titrant. End point is detected by using an indicator or by potentiometric method.

Assay of Ephedrine Hydrochloride Tablets

Procedure : Weigh accurately 20 tablets and grind to fine powder. Weigh accurately a quantity of powder equivalent to about 0.15 g of ephedrine hydrochloride and add glacial acetic acid (30 ml), mercuric acetate solution (10 ml) and crystal-violet solution (0.1 ml). Warm gently the solution, cool and titrate with 0.1 N perchloric acid until the violet colour changes to green blue. Perform a blank titration in the same way.

Ephedrine HCl is too weakly basic to react quantitatively with acetous perchloric acid. Addition of mercuric acetate (which is undissociated in acetic acid solution) to halide salt replaces ion by an equivalent quantity of acetate ion which is a strong base in acetic acid and can react quantitatively with perchloric acid.

$$2C_{10}H_{15}NO.HCl \rightleftharpoons 2C_{10}H_{16}N^{+}O + 2\ Cl^{-}$$

Ephedrine hydrochloride

$$(CH_3COO)_2\ Hg\ (\text{undissociated}) + 2Cl^{-} \longrightarrow HgCl_2 + CH_3COO^{-}$$

Mercuric acetate

$$2CH_3COO^{-} + 2CH_3COOH \longrightarrow CH_3COOH$$

Factor : Each ml of 0.1 N perchloric acid is equivalent to 0.02017 g of $C_{10}H_{15}NO$. HCl.

Alkalimetry

Week acids can be determined by titration with metallic alkoxides using a protophilic solvent. End point can be detected by using indicator or by potentiometric method. For example, barbiturates are weak acid and cannot be estimated in the aqueous solution. They can be estimated by titration with standard sodium methoxide in dimethyl formamide by using thymol blue as indîcator or in pyridine solution. The lithium methoxide solution is preferred over sodium or potassium methoxide which tend to give gelatinous precipitate.

Similarly, supha drugs can also be titrated in dimethylformamide or pyridine or ethylenediamine by standard sodium methoxide.

Assay of Chlorothiazide (B.P. Method)

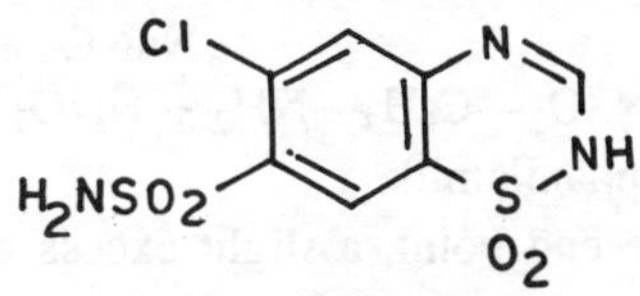

Procedure : Dissolve chlorothiazide ($C_7H_6ClN_3O_4S_2$) (0.25 g) in dimethylformamide (50 ml) and titrate with 0.1 M tetrabutyl ammonium hydroxide and determine the end point potentiometrically at the first inflection. Repeat the operation without the substance being examined. The difference between the titration represents the amount of tetrabutyl ammonium hydroxide required.

Factor : Each ml of 0.1 M tetra-ammonium hydroxide is equivalent to 0.029578 g of $C_7H_6ClN_3O_4S_2$.

Assay of Diphenylhydantoin

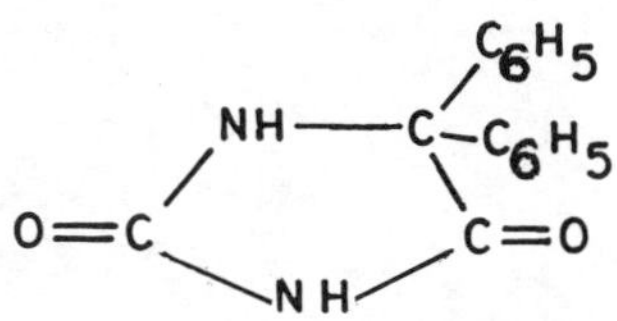

Procedure : Dissolve diphenylhydantoin ($C_{15}H_{12}N_2O_2$) (0.5 g) in dimethyl formamide, add 3 drops of saturated solution of azo violet in benzene and titrate with 0.1 N sodium methoxide to a blue end point. Perform a blank determination and make any necessary correction.

Factor : Each ml of 0.1 N sodium methoxide solution is equivalent to 0.02523 g of $C_{15}H_{12}N_2O_2$.

DIAZOTIZATION

The substances containing primary aromatic amino group are converted into their respective diazonium salts by titration with sodium nitrite at low temperature in the presence of hydrochloric acid.

$$Ar\,NH_2 + Na\,NO_2 \xrightarrow[0-5°C]{HCl} Ar\,N \equiv N^+\,Cl^- + NaCl + 2H_2O$$

Diazonium salt

At the end point, a drop of nitrous acid (formed from $NaNO_2$ in acid medium) reacts with starch iodide paper and gives blue colour due to liberation of iodine.

$$2I^- + 2HNO_2 + 2H^- \longrightarrow I_2 + 2NO\uparrow + 2H_2O$$

$$I_2 \xrightarrow{\text{starch mucilage}} \text{Blue colour}$$

Assay of Sulphanilamide

Procedure : An accurately weighed sample of sulphamilamide (1 g), previouly dried at 105° for 2 hours, is dissolved in concentrated hydrochloric acid (40 ml) and water (100 ml). The solution is cooled to about 5° and titrated with 0.1 M sodium nitrate with the tip of burette well under the surface. The sodium nitrite is added slowly until an immediate blue colour is obtained on adding a drop of the solution to a starch-iodide paper. The end point should be reproducible for a period of atleast 1 minute.

Nitrous acid is formed from sodium nitrite in acidic medium which diazotises sulphanilamide to form the diazonium salt.

$$NaNO_2 + HCl \longrightarrow HNO_2 + NaCl$$

$$\underset{\text{Sulphanilamide}}{H_2NSO_2—C_6H_4—NH_2} + HNO_2 + HCl \longrightarrow H_2NSO_2—C_6H_4—N_2Cl + 2H_2O$$

At the end point, a slight excess of nitrous acid reacts with starch iodide paper to give the blue colour.

Factor : Each ml of 0.1 M $NaNO_2$ is equivalent to 0.01722 g of sulphanilamide.

4

Gravimetric Analysis

Gravimetric analysis is the measurement of weight of a substance in a sample or calculation of weight of a substance from the weight of chemically equivalent amount of some other substance.

In the general reaction, the weight A + B $\longrightarrow$ C + D of either reactant A or B can be calculated from the weight of either product C or D. For example, in the assay of sodium chloride,

$$NaCl + AgNO_3 \longrightarrow AgCl + NaNO_3$$

The silver nitrate is added to precipitate the soluble chloride as insoluble silver chloride which is collected, washed and dried to a constant weight. From the weight of silver chloride, weight of sodium chloride is calculated.

Sometime in the simple gravimetric method, the organic compound is extracted by suitable a solvent from a mixture. The solvent is removed by evaporation/distillation and the residue so obtained is dried to a constant weight.

Gravimetric methods are not in use due to lack of accuracy. They are time consuming in comparison to volumetric methods. Some examples of gravimetrical assays official in I.P. 1966 are illustrated here.

Assay of Sodium Sulphate

Sodium sulphate contains not less than 99% and not more than the equivalent of 100.5% of Na_2SO_4 calculated with reference to the substance dried to a constant weight at 105°.

Weigh accurately about 0.5 g and dissolve in water (100 ml), add hydrochloric acid (1 ml), heat to boiling, add slowly a slight excess of hot solution of barium chloride and heat for half an hour on a water bath. Collect the precipitate, wash and ignite to a constant weight.

Sodium sulphate is precipitated by adding barium chloride solution as insoluble barium sulphate which is filtered and washed with water till filtrate is free from chloride. The precipitate is ignited to a constant weight.

$$\underset{142\ g}{Na_2SO_4} + BaCl_2 \longrightarrow \underset{233.4\ g}{BaSO_4} + 2NaCl$$

Factor : Each g of the residue is equivalent to 0.6085 g of Na_2SO_4.

Assay of Magnesium Sulphate

Magnesium sulphate contains not less than 99.5% $MgSO_4$ calculated with reference to the substance dried to a constant weight at 300°C.

Weigh accurately 0.5 g, dissolve in water (50 ml), add hydrochloric acid (10 ml) and dilute with water (150 ml). Cool to 0°, add solution of ammonium phosphate (25 ml) and slowly with constant stirring dilute ammonia solution until the solution is just alkaline to phenol red. Add a further dilute ammonia solution (10 ml). Stir well, allow to stand for four hours and filter. Wash the precipitate with a mixture of 1 volume of dilute ammonia solution and 19 volumes of water, dissolve the precipitate in 1 N hydrochloric acid (50 ml) and wash the filtrate with hot 0.1 N hydrochloric acid. Combine the solution and washings and dilute to 150 ml with water, add solution of ammonium phosphate (2 ml), add dilute ammonia solution until the solution is just alkaline to a solution of phenol red. Add a further dilute ammonia solution (10 ml), stir well and allow to stand for four hours and filter. Wash the precipitate with a mixture of 1 volume of dilute ammonia solution and 19 volumes of water until free from chloride, dry and ignite to a constant weight at 1100°C.

Magnesium sulphate is precipitated as hydrated magnesium ammonium phosphate, $MgNH_4PO_4 \cdot 6H_2O$ by addition of a solution of ammonium phosphate to an ice cold, acidified solution. The solution is then neutralized by addition of ammonia solution and made alkaline by adding an excess amount of the solution. The solution is allowed to stand for four hours, filtered and the precipitate washed with dilute ammonia. The precipitate is redissolved in hydrochloric acid, reprecipitated as above, collected, washed until free from chloride, dried and ignited. On ignition, magnesium ammonium phosphate is converted to magnesium pyrophosphate which is weighed.

$$\underset{\text{Magnesium ammonium sulphate}}{2MgNH_4PO_4} \longrightarrow \underset{\text{Magnesium pyrophosphate}}{Mg_2P_2O_7} + 2NH_3 + H_2O$$

Factor : Each gram of the residue is equivalent to 1.082 g of $MgSO_4$.

Assay of Zinc Sulphate

Zinc sulphate contains not less than 55.6% and not more than 61% of $ZnSO_4$, corresponding to not less than 99.5% and not more than 102% of the hydrated salt, $ZnSO_4.7H_2O$.

Weigh accurately zinc sulphate (1 g) and dissolve in water (100 ml). Heat the solution to about 90° and add solution of sodium carbonate to precipitate all the zinc, taking care to avoid a large excess of sodium carbonate. Boil for about five minutes and set aside to allow the precipitate to subside. Collect the precipitate in a tared Gooch crucible and wash with water until free from alkali. Dry the residue, ignite and weigh.

Zinc sulphate is precipitated as zinc carbonate by adding sodium carbonate solution.

$$ZnSO_4 + Na_2CO_3 \longrightarrow ZnCO_3\uparrow + Na_2SO_4$$

The precipitate of zinc carbonate is converted to zinc oxide by ignition. The constant weight of zinc oxide is correlated with the weight of zinc sulphate.

$$ZnCO_3 \longrightarrow ZnO + CO_2$$

Factor : Each gram of the residue is equivalent to 1.984 g of $ZnSO_4$.

5

Identification Tests for Cations and Anions

IDENTIFICATION REACTIONS

The following tests may be used for the identification of chemicals referred in the Pharmacopoetia. They are not intended to be applicable to mixtures of substances unless so specified.

Acetates

1. The substance is heated with an equal quantity of *oxalic acid*. Acid vapours with the characteristic odour of acetic acid are liberated.

$$CH_3COONa + (COOH)_2 \longrightarrow CH_3COOH + Na_2CO_3$$

2. The substance (1 g) is warmed with *sulphuric acid* (1 ml) and *alcohol* (3 ml). Ethyl acetate. recognisable by its odour, is evolved (estrification reaction).

$$C_2H_5OH + CH_3COOH \xrightarrow{H_2SO_4} CH_3COOC_2H_5 + H_2O$$

3. The substance (30 mg) is dissolved in water solution (3 ml) lanthanum nitrate, $La(NO_3)_3$ solution (0.25 ml), 0.1 N iodine (0.1 ml) and dilute ammonia solution (0.05 ml) are added in succession and heated carefully to boiling. Within a few minutes, a blue precipitate is formed or a dark blue colour develops.

$$RCOOC_2H_5 + La(NO_3)_3 + I_2 + NH_4OH \longrightarrow \text{Blue ppt}$$

4. The substance (20 mg) is heated with calcium oxide (50 mg); acetone is evolved, which may be detected by the indigo blue colour obtained when vapours impinge on filter paper which has been moistened with a 2 per cent w/v solution of 2-nitrobenzaldehyde in alcohol, dried, and moistened with *N sodium hydroxide*.

$$Ca(CH_3COO)_2 \xrightarrow{\text{heat}} CH_3COCH_3 + CaCO_3$$

Aluminium

1. The substance (20 mg) is dissolved in water (2 ml); 2 N hydrochloric acid (0.5 ml) and thioacetamide reagent (0.5 ml) are added, no precipitate forms. 2 N sodium hydroxide solution is added dropwise; a gelatinous white precipitate appears that re-dissolves on

addition of further sodium hydroxide solution. Gradually ammonium chloride solution is added; the gelatinous white precipitate re-appears.

$$Al^{3+} + 3OH^- \longrightarrow Al(OH)_3 \downarrow$$

2. The substance (20 mg) is dissolved in water (5 ml), five drops of ammonium acetate solution and five drops of a 0.1 per cent w/v solution of mordant blue 3 are added; an intense purple colour is produced.

$Al^{3+} + CH_3COONH_4 +$

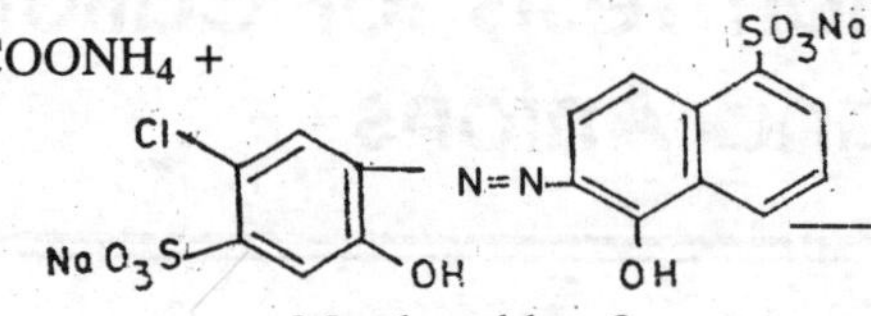

$\longrightarrow$ Purple coloured complex

Mordant blue 3

3. To a solution of the substance in water, dilute ammonia solution is added until a faint precipitate is produced, and then a freshly prepared 0.05 per cent w/v solution of quinalizarin (0.25 ml) in a 1 per cent w/v solution of sodium hydroxide is added, heated to boiling, cooled, and acidified with an excess of acetic acid; a reddish-violet colour is produced.

$$Al^{3+} + 3NH_3 + 3H_2O \longrightarrow Al(OH)_3 \downarrow + 3NH_4^+$$

$$Al(OH)_3 + \text{Quinalizarin} + NaOH \longrightarrow \text{Reddish-violet colour}$$

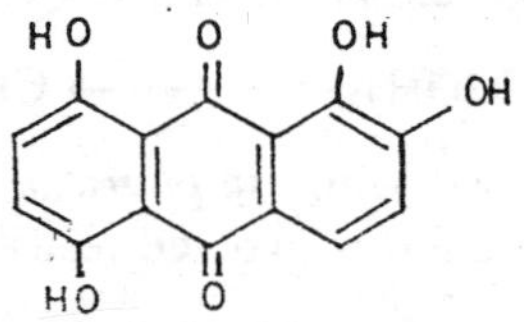

(Quinalizarin)

Ammonium Salts

1. A few mg of the substance are heated with sodium hydroxide solution; ammonia is evolved, which is recognisable by its odour and by its action on moist red litmus paper.

$$NH_4^+ + {}^-OH \longrightarrow NH_3 \downarrow + H_2O$$

2. To the prescribed solution, light magnesium oxide (0.2 g) is added. A current of air is passed through the mixture and the gas, that is evolved, directed to just beneath the surface of a mixture of 0.1 N hydrochloric acid (1 ml) and methyl red solution (0.05 ml); the colour of the solution changes to yellow. On addition of freshly prepared 10 per cent w/v solution of sodium cobaltinitrite (1 ml), a yellow precipitate forms.

$$Na_3[Co(NO_2)_6] + NH_4^+ \longrightarrow (NH_4)_3[CO(NO_2)_6] \downarrow$$

Sodium cobaltinitrite — Yellow precipitate

Antimony

The substance (10 mg) is dissolved with gentle heating in a solution of sodium potassium tartrate (0.5 g) in water (10 ml) and allowed to cool. To this solution (2 ml), sodium sulphide solution is added dropwise, a reddish-orange precipitate is formed which dissolves on adding dilute sodium hydroxide solution.

$$Sb_2S_3 + 8OH^- \longrightarrow 2[Sb(OH)_4]^- + 2SbS_2^-$$

$$Sb_2S_5 + 6OH^- \longrightarrow \underset{\text{Soluble}}{\overset{\text{Soluble}}{SbS_4^{2-}}} + \underset{\text{Soluble}}{\overset{\text{Soluble}}{SbO_3S^{2-}}} + 3H_2O$$

$$2Sb^{3+} + 3S^{2-} \xrightarrow{Na_2S} Sb_2S_3 \downarrow \text{ (antimony sulphide)}$$

Orange red ppt

$$2Sb^{5+} + 5S^{2-} \xrightarrow{Na_2S} Sb_2S_5 \downarrow$$

$$\underset{\text{Sodium potassium tartrate}}{Sb_2O_3/Sb_2O_5 + 2C_4H_4O_6^{2-}} \xrightarrow{Na_2S} \underset{\text{Reddish-orange precipitate.}}{2[(SbO)(C_4H_4O_6)]^-}$$

Arsenic

The prescribed solution (5 ml) is heated on a water-bath with an equal volume of hypophosphorus reagent; a brown precipitate is formed.

Barium

1. Barium salt impart a yellowish-green colour to a non-luminous flame, appearing blue when viewed through green glass.
2. The substance (20 mg) is dissolved in dilute hydrochloric acid (5 ml), dilute sulphuric acid (2 ml) added; a white precipitate forms which is insoluble in nitric acid.

$$Ba^{2+} + SO_4^{2-} \xrightarrow{HCl} BaSO_4 \downarrow$$

Benzoates

1. To a 10 per cent w/v neutral solution (1 ml), ferric chloride test solution (0.5 ml) is added; a dull-yellow precipitate, soluble in solvent ether, is formed.

$$3C_6H_5COO^- + 2Fe^{3+} + 3H_2O \longrightarrow \underset{\text{Dull-yellow ppt.}}{Fe(C_6H_5COO)_3 \,.\, Fe(OH)_3 \downarrow} + H_2O$$

2. Ths substance (0.2 g) is moistened with sulphuric acid and the bottom of the tube warmed gently; a white sublimate is deposited on the inner walls of the tube and no charring occurs.

$$2C_6H_5COONa + H_2SO_4 \xrightarrow{Heat} \text{White sublimate}$$

3. The substance (0.5 g) is dissolved in water (10 ml), and hydrochloric acid (0.5 ml) added. The precipitate obtained, after crystallization from water and drying under reduced pressure, melts at about 122°.

$$C_6H_5COONa + HCl \longrightarrow \underset{\text{Benzoic acid}}{C_6H_5COOH} + NaCl$$

Bicarbonates

1. Solutions of bicarbonates, when boiled, liberate carbon dioxide.

$$2NaHCO_3 \xrightarrow{\text{Heat}} Na_2CO_3 + H_2O + CO_2 \downarrow$$

2. A solution of the substance is treated with a solution of magnesium sulphate; no precipitate is formed (distinction from carbonates). On boiling, a white precipitate is formed.

$$2Na_2HCO_3 \xrightarrow{\text{Heat}} Na_2CO_3 + H_2O + CO_2$$
$$Na_2CO_3 + H_2O \rightleftharpoons 2Na + 2OH^- + CO_2$$
$$MgSO_4 + OH^- \rightleftharpoons MgOH + SO_4^{2-}$$
$$2MgOH^+ + CO_2 \rightleftharpoons \underset{\text{White ppt}}{Mg(OH)_2 \downarrow} + CO_3^{2-}$$

3. The substance (0.1 g) is suspended in water (2 ml) in a test tube; 2 N acetic acid (2 ml) is added. The tube is closed immediately using a stopper fitted with a glass tube bent at two right-angles, heated gently and the gas collected in barium hydroxide solution (5 ml); a white precipitate forms that dissolves on addition of an excess of dilute hydrochloric acid.

$$NaHCO_3 + CH_3COOH \longrightarrow CH_3COONa + H_2O + CO_2$$
$$Ba(OH)_2 + CO_2 \longrightarrow BaCO_3 \downarrow + H_2O$$
$$BaCO_3 + 2HCl \longrightarrow BaCl_2 + CO_2 \uparrow + H_2O$$

Bismuth

1. To the substance, 2 N hydrochloric acid (10 ml) is added, headed to boiling for one minute, cooled and filtered, if necessary. To 1 ml of the solution obtained, water (20 ml) is added; a white or slightly yellow precipitate appears which on addition of 0.05 to 0.1 ml of sodium sulphide solution turns brown.

$$Bi^{3+} + 3HCl \longrightarrow BiCl_3 + 3H^+$$
$$BiCl_3 + 4H_2O \longrightarrow Bi(OH)_3 + H_3O^+ + 2Cl^-$$
$$Bi(OH)_2Cl \longrightarrow BiOCl + H_2O$$

Bismuth oxychloride (White ppt.)

$$2BiO^+ + 3HS^- + H^+ \longrightarrow Bi_2S_3 \downarrow + 2H_2O$$

2. To the substance (50 mg), 2 N nitric acid (10 ml) is added, heated to boiling for one minute, allowed to cool and filtered, if necessary. To 5 ml of the solution obtained, 10 per cent w/v solution of thiourea (2 ml) is added; an orange yellow colour or an orange precipitate is produced. a 2.5 per cent w/v solution of sodium fluoride (4 ml) is added; the solution is not decoulourized within thirty minutes.

$$Bi^{3+} + 3HNO_3 \longrightarrow Bi(NO_3)_3 + 3H^+$$
$$Bi(NO_3)_3 + NH_2CSNH_2 \longrightarrow \text{Orange yellow ppt.}$$

Bromides

1. A quantity of the substance, equivalent to about 3 mg of bromide ion, is dissolved in water (2 ml). It is acidified with 2 N nitric acid and 0.1 N silver nitrate (1 ml) added, shaked and allowed to stand; a curdy, pale-yellow precipitate forms. The precipitate is centrifuged and washed rapidly with three quantities in subdued light. The precipitate is suspended in water (2 ml) and 10 N ammonia (1.5 ml) is added; the precipitate dissolves with difficulty.

$$NaBr + AgNO_3 \longrightarrow AgBr + NaNO_3$$

2. About 10 mg are dissolved in water (2 ml) and chlorine solution (1 ml) is added; bromine is evolved, which is soluble in two or three drops of chloroform, forming a reddish solution. The addition of phenol solution to the aqueous solution containing liberated bromine yields a white precipitate.

$$2KBr + Cl_2 \longrightarrow 2KCl + Br_2$$

$$\underset{\text{Phenol}}{C_6H_5OH} + 3Br_2 \longrightarrow \underset{\substack{\text{Tribromophenol} \\ \text{(White ppt.)}}}{C_6H_2(Br)_3OH} + 3HBr$$

Note : *In testing for bromides in the presence of iodides, all iodine must first be removed by boiling the aqueous solution with an excess of lead dioxide.*

Calcium

1. The substance (20 mg) is dissolved in 5 M acetic acid (5 ml). Potassium ferrocyanide solution (10.5 ml) is added; the solution remains clear. On addition of ammonium chloride (50 mg), a white crystalline precipitate is formed.

$$Ca^{2+} + 2K^+ + [Fe(CN)_6]^{4-} \longrightarrow CaK_2[Fe(CN)]_6 \downarrow$$

2. To a solution of the substance, a few drops of a solution of ammonium oxalate are added; a white precipitate is obtained that is only sparingly soluble in dilute acetic acid but is soluble in hydrochloric acid.

$$(NH_4)_2C_2O_4 \rightleftharpoons 2NH_4^+ + C_2O_4^{2-}$$

$$Ca^{2+} + C_2O_4^{2-} \longrightarrow \underset{\substack{\text{Calcium oxalate} \\ \text{White ppt.}}}{CaC_2O_4 \downarrow}$$

$$CaC_2O_4 + 2HCl \longrightarrow CaCl_2 + (COOH)_2$$

3. The substance (20 mg) is dissolved in the minimum quantity of dilute hydrochloric acid and neutralized with dilute sodium hydroxide solution: ammonium carbonate solution (5 ml); a white precipitate is formed which, after boiling and cooling the mixture, is only sparingly soluble in ammonium chloride solution.

$$CaCl_2 + (NH_4)_2CO_3 \longrightarrow 2NH_4Cl + CaCO_3 \downarrow$$

$$Ba(OH)_2 + CO_2 \longrightarrow \underset{\text{White ppt}}{BaCO_3 \downarrow} H_2O$$

$$BaCO_3 + 2HCl \longrightarrow BaCl_2 \downarrow + CO_2 \uparrow + H_2O$$

2. A solution of the substance is treated with a solution of magnesium sulphate; a white precipitate is formed (distinction from bicarbonates).

$$5Mg^{2+} + 5CO_3^{2-} + 6H_2O \longrightarrow \underset{\text{White precipitate}}{MgCO_3 . Mg(OH)_2 . 5H_2O} \downarrow + CO_2 \uparrow$$

Chlorides

1. A quantity of the substance equivalent to about 2 mg of chloride ion is dissolved in water (2 ml). It is acidified with dilute nitric acid and silver nitrate solution (0.5 ml) added. The solution is shaken and allowed to stand; a curdy white precipitate is formed, which is insoluble in nitric acid, but soluble, after being well washed with water, in dilute ammonia solution, from which it is re-precipitated by the addition of nitric acid.

$$NaCl + AgNO_3 \longrightarrow AgCl \downarrow + NaNO_3$$

$$AgCl + 2NH_3 \longrightarrow \underset{\text{Soluble complex}}{Ag(NH_3)_2^+ Cl^-}$$

$$Ag(NH_3)_2^+ Cl^- + HNO_3 \longrightarrow AgCl \downarrow + (NH_4)_2NO_3$$

2. A quantity of the substance equivalent to about 10 mg of chloride ion is introduced into a test-tube; potassium dichromate (0.2 g and sulphuric acid (1 ml) are added. A filter-paper strip moistened with diphenylcarbazide solution is placed over the opening of the test-tube; the paper turns violet-red. The moistened paper is not brought into contact with the potassium dichromate solution.

$$K_2Cr_2O_7 + 4NaCl + 6H_2SO_4 \longrightarrow \underset{\text{Chromyl chloride}}{2CrO_2Cl_2} + 2KHSO_4 + 4NaHSO_4 + 3H_2O$$

$$CrO_2Cl_2 + \underset{\text{(Diphenylcarbazide)}}{C_6H_5NHNHCONHNHC_6H_5} + H_2O \longrightarrow \text{Violet red colour}$$

Citrates

1. To a neutral solution of the substance, a solution of calcium chloride is added, no precipitate is produced. The solution is boiled, a white precipitate, soluble in acetic acid, formed.

$$2Na_3C_6H_5O_7 + 3CaCl_2 + 4H_2O \longrightarrow Ca_3(C_6H_5O_7) . 4H_2O \downarrow + 6NaCl$$

2. A quantity of the substance is dissolved in water (5 ml). Sulphuric acid (0.5 ml) and potassium permanganate solutions (3 ml) are added. It is warmed until the colour of the permangnate solution is discharged and 10% w/v solution of sodium nitroprusside added in 2 N sulphuric acid and 4 g of sulphamic acid, make alkaline with strong ammonia solution, further addition of strong ammonia solution produces a violet colour, turning to violet-blue.

$$\underset{\text{Citric acid}}{C(CH_2COOH)_2 (OH) COOH} + KMnO_4 \longrightarrow \underset{\text{Acetone dicarboxylic acid}}{CO(CH_2COOH)_2}$$

$$CO(CH_2COOH)_2 + Na_2[Fe(CN)_5NO] + H_2SO_4 + H_2N\text{–}SO_3H + NH_3 \longrightarrow \text{Violet colour}$$

Ferric Salts

1. A quantity of the substance equivalent to about 10 mg of iron is dissolved in water (1 ml). A 5 per cent w/v solution of potassium ferrocyanide (1 ml) is added; an intense blue precipitate is formed which is insoluble in dilute hydrochloric acid.

$$4FeCl_3 + 3K_4Fe(CN)_6 \longrightarrow Fe_4[Fe(CN)_6]_3 \downarrow + 12\ KCl$$

Potassium ferrocyanide — Blue colour

2. To 3 ml of a solution containing about 0.1 mg of iron, 3 N hydrochloric acid (1 ml) and ammonium thicyanate solution (1 ml) are added; the solution becomes blood-red in colour. Two portions, each of 1 ml of the mixture, are taken. To one portion solvent ether (5 ml) is added, shaked and allowed to stand; the ether layer becomes pink. To the other portion 0.2 M mercuric chloride (3 ml) is added; the red colour disappears.

$$FeCl_3 + 3NH_4SCN \longrightarrow Fe(SCN)_3 + NH_4Cl$$

Ferric tiocyanate (Red colour)

$$2Fe(SCN)_3 + 3HgCl \longrightarrow 3Hg(SCN)_2 + 2FeCl_3$$

Mercuric thiocyanate (Colourless)

3. To 2 ml of a solution containing about 0.1 mg of iron, acetic acid is added until the solution is strongly acidic. A 0.2 per cent solution of 8-hydroxy-7-iodoquinoline-5-sulphonic acid (2 ml) is added. A stable green coloured complex is produced.

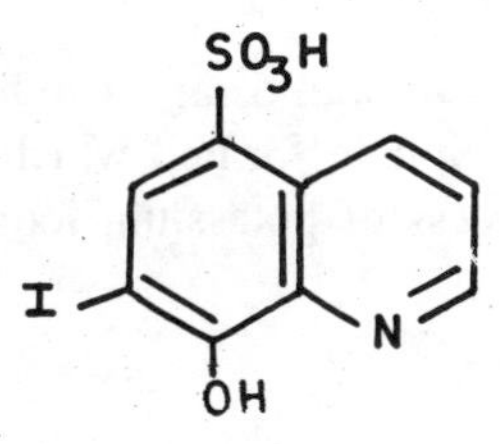

8-Hydroxy-7-isoquinoline, 5-sulphonic acid

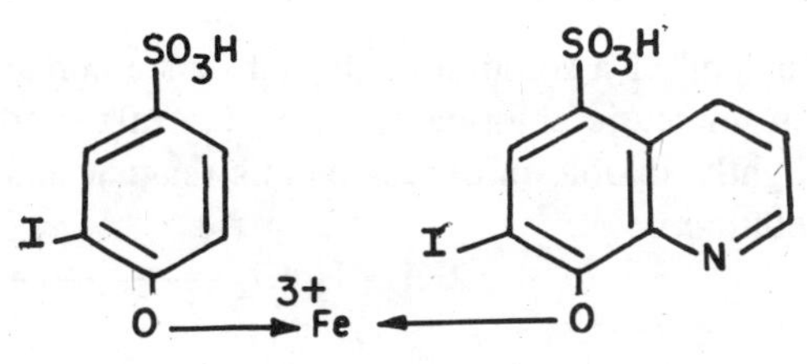

Green coloured complex

Ferrous Salts

1. A quantity of the substance corresponding to about 10 mg of iron is dissolved in water (2 ml). To it dilute sulphuric acid (2 ml) and 0.1 per cent solution of 1, 10-phenanthroline (1 ml) are added. An intense red colour is produced; the colour is discharged by addition of a slight excess of 0.1 N ceric ammonium sulphate.
2. To 1 ml of a solution of iron, potassium ferricyanide solution (1 ml) is added; a dark blue precipitate is formed that is insoluble in dilute hydrochloric acid and is decomposed by sodium hydroxide solution.

$$Fe^{++} + 2K^{+} + [Fe(CN)_6]^{4-} \longrightarrow K_2Fe[Fe(CN)_6] \downarrow$$

3. To 1 ml of a solution containing not less than 1 mg of iron, potassium ferrocyanide solution (1 ml) is added; a white precipitate is formed which rapidly becomes blue and is insoluble in dilute hydrochloric acid.

$$2FeSO_4 + K_4Fe(CN)_6 \longrightarrow \underset{\text{Ferrous ferrocyanide (White ppt)}}{Fe_2[Fe(CN)_6]^{+}} \,.\, 2K_2SO_4$$

$$\downarrow [O], \text{ Air}$$

$$\underset{\text{Persion blue}}{Fe_4[Fe(CN)_6]_3}$$

Iodides

1. A quantity of the substance equivalent to about 4 mg of iodide ion is dissolved in water (2 ml). It is acidified with dilute nitric acid and silver nitrate (0.5 ml) solution is added. It is shaken and allowed to stand, a curdy pale-yellow precipitate forms. It is centrifuged and the precipitate washed rapidly with three quantities, each of 1 ml of water in subdued light. The precipitate is suspended in water (2 ml) and 10 N ammonia (1.5 ml) is added; the precipitate does not dissolve.

$$NaI + AgNO_3 \xrightarrow{HNO_3} \underset{\text{Yellow}}{AgI} \downarrow + NaNO_3$$

2. To 0.2 ml of a solution of the substance containing the equivalent of about 5 mg of iodide ion per ml., 2 N sulphuric acid (0.5 ml), potassium dichromate solution (0.15 ml), water (2 ml) and chloroform (2 ml) are added. It is shaked for a few seconds and allowed to stand; the violet or violet-red colour appears in the chloroform layer.

$$Cr_2O_7^{2-} + 6I^{-} + 14H^{+} \longrightarrow 2Cr^{3+} + 7H_2O + 2I_2 \text{ (violet)}$$

3. To 1 ml of a solution of the substance containing the equivalent of about 5 mg of iodide ion, mercuric chloride solution (0.5 ml) is added; a dark red precipitate formed which is slightly soluble in excess of this reagent and very soluble in excess of potassium iodide solution.

$$2KI + HgCl_2 \longrightarrow \underset{\text{Mercuric iodide (red)}}{HgI_2} \downarrow + 2KCl$$

$$HgI_2 + 2KI \longrightarrow \underset{\text{(Potassium mercuri-iodide)}}{K_2HgI}$$

Lactates

A mixture of aqueous solution of the substance, bromine water and 2 N sulphuric acid is heated on a water-bath until the colour is discharged. After addition of ammonium sulphate, sodium nitroprusside solution (10%) in 2 N sulphuric acid is added. Strong ammonium solution is mixed and left for 30 minutes. A dark green ring appears at the junction of two layers.

Lead

1. The substance (0.1 g) is dissolved in dilute acetic acid (1 ml). To it, potassium chromate solution (2 ml) is added; a yellow precipitate forms which is insoluble in sodium hydroxide solution.

$$Pb^{2+} + CrO_4^{2-} \longrightarrow PbCrO_4 \downarrow$$

(Lead chromate)

$$PbCl_2 + K_2CrO_4 \longrightarrow PbCrO_4 \downarrow + 2KCl$$

2. The substance (50 mg) is dissolved in dilute acetic acid (1 ml). To it, water (10 ml) and potassium iodide solution (0.2 ml) are added; a yellow precipitate forms. The mixture is heated to boiling for one or two minutes, and allowed to cool; the precipitate is re-formed as glistening, yellow plates.

$$Pb^{2+} + 2I^- \longrightarrow PbI_2$$

$$Pb(NO_3)_2 + 2KI \longrightarrow PbI_2 \downarrow + 2KNO_3$$

Yellow ppt.

Magnesium

1. The substance (15 mg) is dissolved in water (2 ml). To it, dilute ammonia solution (1 ml) is added; a white precipitate forms that is re-dissolved by additing 2 M ammonium chloride solution (1 ml). To the solution 0.25 M disodium hydrogen phosphate (1 ml) is added; a white crystalline precipitate forms.
Ammonium chloride prevents precipitation of magnesium hydroxide due to suppression of dissociation of ammonium hydroxide caused by a common ion effect.

$$NH_4Cl \longrightarrow NH_4^+ + Cl^-$$

$$NH_4OH \longrightarrow NH_4^+ + OH^-$$

$$Mg^{2+} + OH^- \longrightarrow Mg(OH)_2 \downarrow$$

$$Mg^{2+} + NH_4^+ + PO_4^{3-} + 6H_2O \longrightarrow MgNH_4PO_4 \,.\, 6H_2O \downarrow$$

White ppt

$$MgSO_4 + Na_2HPO_4 + NH_4OH + 6H_2O \longrightarrow MgNH_4PO_4 \,.\, 6H_2O \downarrow + Na_2SO_4 + H_2O$$

2. To 0.5 ml of a neutral or slightly acidic solution of the substance, a 0.1 per cent solution (0.2 ml) of titan yellow and 0.1 N sodium hydroxide (0.5 ml) are added; a bright red turbidity develops which gradually settles to give a bright red precipitate.

Nitrates

1. To the substance (15 mg) dissolved in water (0.5 ml), sulphuric acid (1 ml) is added. Then it is mixed and cooled. The tube is inclined and without mixing, ferrous sulphate solution (0.5 ml) is added. A brown colour forms at the interface of the two liquids.

$$3Fe^{2+} + 4H^+ + NO^{3-} \longrightarrow NO + 3Fe^{3+} + 2H_2O$$

$$Fe^{2+} + NO \longrightarrow [Fe(NO)]^{2+} \text{ (Brown colour)}$$

2. A mixture of nitrobenzene. (0.1 ml), sulphuric acid (0.2 ml) and powdered substance is allowed to stand for five minutes and cooled in ice water whilst adding slowly with stirring water (5 ml) and then sodium hydroxide solution (5 ml). To it, acetone (5 ml) is added, shaked, and allowed to stand; the upper layer shows an intense violet colour.

Phosphates (Orthophosphates)

1. To 5 ml of the prescribed solution, neutralized to pH 7.0, silver nitrate solution is added; a light yellow precipitate forms, the colour of which is not changed by boiling and which is readily soluble in dilute ammonia solution and in dilute nitric acid.

$$3Ag^+ + 2HPO_4^{2-} \longrightarrow Ag_3PO_4 \downarrow + H_2PO_4^-$$

$$Ag_3PO_4 \longrightarrow 3Ag^+ + PO_4^{3-}$$

$$Ag^+ + 2NH_3 \rightleftharpoons [Ag(NH_3)_2]^+$$

Silver diamino complex soluble

$$PO_4^{3-} + H_2O \longrightarrow HOP_4^{2-} + OH^-$$

$$OH^- + H^+ \xrightarrow{HNO_3} H_2O$$

2. The prescribed solution (1 ml) is mixed with ammonical magnesium sulphate solution (1 ml); a white crystalline precipitate is produced.

$$Mg^{2+} + HPO_4^{2-} + NH_3 + 6H_2O \longrightarrow MgNH_4PO_4 \cdot 6H_2O$$

3. To 2 ml of the prescribed solution, dilute nitric acid (2 ml) and ammonium molybdate solution (4 ml) are added and then solution warmed; a bright canary-yellow precipitate is formed.

$$12MoO_4^{2-} + HPO_4^{2-} + 3NH_4^+ + 23H^+ \longrightarrow (NH_4)_3[P(Mo_{12}O_{40})] + 12H_2O$$

Ammonium phosphomolybdate (Canary-yellow)

Potassium

1. The substance (50 mg) is dissolved in water (1 ml). To it, dilute acetic acid (1 ml) and freshly prepared 10 per cent solution of sodium cobaltinitrite (1 ml) are added; a yellow or orange-yellow precipitate forms immediately.

$$[Co(NO_2)_6]^{3-} + 3K^+ \longrightarrow K_3[Co(NO_2)_6] \downarrow$$

Potassium cobaltnitrite

2. The substance (0.1 g) is dissolved in water (2 ml). The solution is heated with sodium carbonate solution (1 ml); no precipitate forms. To it, sodium sulphide solution (0.05 ml) is added; no precipitate forms. It is cooled in ice water and 15 per cent w/v solution (2 ml) of tartaric acid is added and then allowed to stand; a white or yellow crystalline precipitate forms.

$$KCl + H_2C_4H_4O_6 \longrightarrow KHC_4H_4O_6 + HCl$$

Yellow ppt

3. A few mg of the substance is ignited, cooled and dissolved in the minimum quantity of water. To this solution, platinic chloride solution (1 ml) is added in the presence of hydrochloric acid (1 ml); a yellow, crystalline precipitate forms, which on ignition leaves a residue of potassium chloride and platinum.

$$H_2[PtCl_6] + 2KCl \longrightarrow \underset{\text{Yellow ppt.}}{K_2[PtCl_6]} + 2\,HCl$$

Salicylates

1. To a neutral solution of the substance, ferric chloride test solution is added. A violet colour is produced which persists after the addition of dilute acetic acid.

$$\underset{\text{Sodium salycylate}}{3C_6H_4(OH)COONa} + FeCl_3 \longrightarrow \underset{\substack{\text{Ferric salicylate}\\\text{(violet)}}}{[C_6H_4(OH)COO]_3Fe} + NaCl$$

2. To an aqueous solution of the substance, hydrochloric acid (0.5 ml) is added. The precipitate is filtered and recrystallized from hot water which melted at 159°C.

$$\underset{\text{Sodium salycylate}}{C_6H_4(OH)COONa} + HCl_3 \longrightarrow \underset{\text{Salicylic acid}}{C_6H_4(OH)COOH\downarrow} + NaCl$$

3. To an aqueous solution of the substance, bromine solution is added. A cream-coloured precipitate is produced.

$$\underset{\text{Sodium salycylate}}{C_6H_4(OH)\,COONa} + Br_2 \xrightarrow{H_2O} \underset{\text{Tribromophenol}}{C_6H_2(OH)\,Br_3}$$

Silver

1. The substance (10 mg) is dissolved in water (10 ml). To it, dilute hydrochloric acid (0.3 ml) is added; a curdy white precipitate, soluble in dilute ammonia solution, is formed. Potassium iodide solution is added; a yellow precipitate is formed.

$$Ag^+ + Cl^- \longrightarrow [Ag(NH_3)_2]^+\,Cl^-$$

$$Ag(NH_3)Cl + KI + 2H_2O \longrightarrow AgI\downarrow + KCl + 2NH_4OH$$

2. The substance (10 mg) is dissolved in water (10 ml) and potassium chromate solution (2 ml) added; a red precipitate, soluble in nitric acid, is formed.

$$2Ag^+ + CrO_4^{2-} \longrightarrow \underset{\text{Red precipitate}}{Ag_2CrO_4\downarrow}$$

Sodium

1. To the substance (0.1 g) dissolved in water (2 ml). 15 per cent solution of potassium carbonate (2 ml) is added and heated to boiling; no precipitate forms. To it, freshly prepared potassium antimonate solution (4 ml) is added and heated to boiling. The solution is allowed to cool in ice water and, if necessary, rubbed the inside of the test-tube with a glass rod; a dense, white precipitate is formed.

$$NaCl + KH_2SbO_4 \longrightarrow NaH_2SbO_4\downarrow + KCl$$

2. A solution of the substance is acidified with N acetic acid and an excess of magnesium uranyl acetate solution added; a yellow crystalline precipitate is formed.

$$Na^+ + Mg^{2+} + 3UO_2^{2+} + 8C_2H_3O_2^- + HC_2H_3O_2 + 9H_2O \longrightarrow NaMg(UO_2)_3(C_2H_3O_2)_9 . 9H_2O + H^+$$

Sulphates

1. To the substance (50 mg) dissolved in 5 ml of water, dilute hydrochloric acid (1 ml) and barium chloride solution (1 ml) are added; a white precipitate forms.

$$Ba^{2+} + SO_4^{2-} \longrightarrow BaSO_4 \downarrow$$

2. The substance (50 mg) dissolved in water (5 ml), lead acetate solution (2 ml) is added; a white precipitate, soluble in ammonium acetate and sodium hydroxide solution, is formed.

$$PbSO_4 + 4C_2H_3O_2^- \longrightarrow [Pb(C_2H_3O_2)_4]^{2-} + SO_4$$

$$PbSO_4 + 3OH^- \longrightarrow HPbO_2^- + H_2O + SO_4^{2-}$$

3. Iodine solution (0.1 ml) is added to the suspension obtained in Test 1; the suspension remains yellow (distinction from sulphites and dithionites) but is decolourized by adding, dropwise stannous chloride solution (distinction from iodates). The mixture is boiled; no coloured precipitate appears (distinction from selenates and tungstates).

Tartrates

1. The substance is warmed with sulphuric acid; charring occurs and carbon monoxide, which burns with blue flame, when ignited, is evolved.

$$H_2C_4H_4O_6 \longrightarrow CO_2 \uparrow + CO \uparrow + 2C + 3H_2O \uparrow$$

$$C + H_2SO_4 \longrightarrow 2SO_2 + CO_2 \uparrow + 2H_2O$$

$$2CO + O_2 \xrightarrow{\text{Blue flame}} 2CO_2$$

2. The substance (20 mg) is dissolved in water (5 ml). To it, 1 per cent solution of ferrous sulphate (0.05 ml) and hydrogen peroxide solution (0.05 ml) are added, a transient yellow colour is produced. A 2N sodium hydroxide solution is added dropwise; an intense blue colour is produced.

$$\begin{matrix} CH(OH)COOH \\ | \\ CH(OH)COOH \end{matrix} + H_2O_2 \longrightarrow \begin{matrix} C(OH)COOH \\ \| \\ C(OH)COOH \end{matrix} + 2H_2O$$

3. A solution (0.1 ml) containing the equivalent of about 2 mg of tartaric acid is heated for five to ten minutes with 10 per cent solution of potassium bromide (0.1 ml), a 2 per cent solution of resorcinol (0.1 ml) and sulphuric acid (3 ml); a dark-blue colour is produced that changes to red when the solution is cooled and poured into water.

Thiosulphates

1. To the substance (0.1 g), dissolved is water (5 ml), add hydrochloric acid (2 ml), a white

precipitate is formed which soon turns yellow and sulphur dioxide is evolved, recognisable by its odour.

$$S_2O_3^{2-} \longrightarrow H_2S_2O_3 + S\downarrow$$

$$H_2S_2O_3 \longrightarrow H_2O + SO_2 + S\downarrow$$

2. To the substance (0.1 g), dissolved in water (2 ml), ferric chloride test solution (2 ml) is added, a dark violet colour is produced which quickly disappears.

$$2S_2O_3 + 3Fe^{3+} \xrightarrow{\text{Neutral}} [Fe(S_2O_{3)_2})_2]^- \longrightarrow 2Fe^+ + S_4O_6^{2-}$$

Ferric thiosulphate complex (Violet colour) — Colourless

$$2FeCl_3 + Na_2S_2O_3 + H_2O \xrightarrow{H^+} 2FeCl_2 + 2NaCl + H_2SO_3 + S$$

$$Na_2S_2O_3 + 2HCl \rightleftharpoons 2NaCl + H_2SO_3 + S$$

$$2H_2SO_3 + 2FeCl_3 \rightleftharpoons Fe_2(SO_4)_3 + 6HCl$$

Ferric sulphate
(Violet colour)

$$Fe_2(SO_3)_3 \longrightarrow FeSO_2 + FeS_2O_6$$

3. Solutions of thiosulphates decolourize iodine solution; the decolourized solutions do not give the reactions of sulphates.

$$2S_2O_3^{2-} + I_2 \longrightarrow 2I^- + [S_4O_6]^{2-}$$

4. Solutions of thiosulphates decolourize bromine solution; the decolourized solutions give the reactions of sulphates.

$$S_2O_3^{2-} + 4Br_2 + 5H_2O \longrightarrow 8Br^- + 10H^+ + 2SO_2^{2-}$$

Zinc

1. The substance (0.1 g) is dissolved in water (5 ml). To it, sodium hydroxide solution (0.2 ml) is added; a white precipitate forms. A further sodium hydroxide solution (2 ml) is added; the precipitate dissolves. Ammonium chloride solution (10 ml) is added; the solution remains clear, but a flocculent white precipitate forms on addition of sodium sulphide solution (0.1 ml).

$$Zn^{2+} + 2OH^- \longrightarrow Zn(OH)_2\downarrow$$

$$ZnCl_2 + 2NaOH \longrightarrow Zn(OH)_2 + NaCl$$

$$Zn(OH)_2 + 2NaOH^- \longrightarrow Na_2ZnO_2 + 2H_2O$$

Sodium zincate

$$Na_2ZnO_2 + H_2S \longrightarrow ZnS\downarrow + 2NaOH$$

White ppt.

2. The substance (0.1 g) is dissolved in water (5 ml), acidified with dilute sulphuric acid, one drop of a 0.1 per cent w/v solution of copper sulphate and ammonium mercuri-thiocyanate solution (2 ml) are added; a violet precipitate is formed.

$$Zn^{2+} + [Hg(SCN)_4]^{2-} \longrightarrow Zn[Hg(SCN)_4]$$

3. The substance (0.1 g) is dissolved in water (5 ml) and potassium ferrocyanide solution (2 ml) added; a white precipitate is formed which is insoluble in dilute hydrochloric acid.

$$2Zn^{2+} + 2K^{+} + 2[Fe(CN)_6]^{4-} \longrightarrow K_2Zn_2[Fe_3(CN_6)_6]_2$$

Potassium zinc ferricyanide
(White ppt.)

6

Identification Tests for Inorganic Substances

Identification tests are performed to determine the quality of a drug so that it can be used with safety. These tests for inorganic drugs are based generally on reactions of an anion or a cation present in a molecule.

Identification tests of some inorganic substances, feasible in the laboratory, are presented in this chapter.

Ammonium Chloride	Iodine
Barium sulphate Boric acid Bentonite	Magnesium sulphate Mercuric oxiide
	Potassium permanganate
Calcium gluconate Chlorinated lime	Sodium benzoate Sodium bicarbonate Sodium chloride Sodium thiosulphate
Ferrous gluconate Ferric ammonium sulphate Ferrous sulphate	Zinc sulphate Zinc oxide
Hydrogen peroxide	

Ammonium Chloride (NH_4Cl)

Ammonium chloride is an expectorant, diuretic and systemic acidifier.

It is available as odourless, colourless or white crystalline powder with saline taste. The salt is freely soluble in water but slightly soluble in alcohol.

Identification Tests : Identification tests are based on characteristics of ammonium and chloride ions.

Test for ammonium ion :

(1) Heat a small amount of ammonium chloride with solution of sodium hydroxide, ammonia gas is evolved. The evolved NH_3 is identified by the following tests:

$$NH_4Cl + NaOH \longrightarrow NH_3 \uparrow + H_2O + NaCl$$

(a) It has a characteristic smell.

(b) Bring a glass rod dipped in conc. hydrochloric acid at the mouth of the test tube. Ammonia gas forms dense white fumes of ammonium chloride.

(c) Bring a wet red litmus paper at the mouth of the test tube. It turns red litmus blue.

(2) Add few drops of sodium cobaltinitrite to ammonium chloride solution. Yellow precipitate of ammonium cobaltinitrite is formed.

$$3NH_3Cl + Na_3\,[CO\,(NO_2)_6] \longrightarrow \underset{\text{Ammonium Cobaltinitrite}}{(NH_4)_3\,[CO\,(NO_2)_6]} + 3\,NH_4NO_3$$

Test for Chloride Ion : Add dilute nitric acid (1 ml) to a solution of ammonium chloride (3 ml). Add few drops of silver nitrate solution, a white precipitate of silver chloride, is formed. On addition of dilute ammonia solution, the precipitate dissolves due to formation of a complex

$$NH_4Cl + AgNO_3 \longrightarrow \underset{\text{Silver chloride}}{AgCl\downarrow} + NH_4\,NO_3$$

$$AgCl + 2\,NH_3 \longrightarrow [Ag\,(NH_3)_2]^+\,Cl^-$$

Barium Sulphate ($BaSO_4$)

It is used as a diagnostic aid. It is a heavy, odourless, tasteless, white fine powder. Barium sulphate is insoluble in water, organic solvents and in dilute solution of acids and of alkalies.

Identification Tests : Identification tests are based on the presence of barium and sulphate ions.

Boil barium sulphate (0.2g) with 50% solution of sodium carbonate (5 ml) for five minutes. Boil the solid mass with hot water and filter. The salt is insoluble. It is converted into less soluble salt by fusion with anhydrous sodium/potassium carbonate. The resulting mass is treated with hot water and filtered. The filtrate is tested for sulphate and the residue is tested for barium

$$BaSO_4 + Na_2\,CO_3 \longrightarrow Na_2\,SO_4 + Ba\,CO_3$$

Tests for Sulphate :

(1) Add barium chloride solution (1 ml) to a part of the filtrate. A white precipitate due to formation of barium sulphate is formed.

$$Na_2SO_4 + BaCl_2 \longrightarrow \underset{\substack{\text{Barious sulphate} \\ \text{(While ppt)}}}{BaSO_4} + 2NaCl$$

(2) Add lead acetate solution (1 ml) to the filtrate (1 ml). A white precipitate of lead sulphate is formed.

$$Na_2\,SO_4 + (CH_3\,COO)_2\,Pb \longrightarrow Pb\,SO_4\downarrow + 2\,CH_3COOH.$$

The precipitate is soluble in ammonium acetate solution and sodium hydroxide solution.

Tests for Barium :

(1) Dissolve a portion of residue in hydrochloric acid and perform flame test. Yellowish-green colour indicates the presence of barium.

(2) Wash the above residue with successive small quantities of water. To the residue add dilute hydrochloric acid (5 ml), filter and to the filtrate, add acid dilute sulphuric acid (0.3 ml). A white precipitate of barium sulphate is formed.

$$BaCO_3 + HCl \longrightarrow BaCl_2 + CO_2 + H_2O$$

$$BaCl_2 + H_2SO_4 \longrightarrow \underset{\text{(White ppt)}}{\underset{\text{Barium sulphate}}{BaSO_4}} + 2HCl$$

Boric acid (H_3BO_3)

Boric acid is a local anti-infective agent. It is mainly used in eye drops and in dusting powders. Boric acid is a colourless or white crystalline powder. It is odourless and taste is slightly acidic and bitter with a sweetish after taste. Boric acid is sparingly soluble in water and alcohol, freely soluble in boiling water, boiling alcohol and glycerine.

Identification Tests

(1) Dissolve 0.1 g by gentle warming with methyl alcohol (5 ml) to which a few drops of sulphuric acid have been added. Ignite the solution, the flame has green border (Flame test). The green colour is due to formation of methyl borate

$$\underset{\text{Boric acid}}{H_3BO_3} + CH_3OH \longrightarrow \underset{\text{Methyl borate}}{B(OCH_3)_3} \uparrow + 3H_2O$$

(2) Dissolve boric acid (3 g) in boiling water (90 ml) and cool. The solution is faintly acidic.

Bentonite

Bentonite, a colloidal hydrated aluminium silicate, is used as a suspending agent. It is odourless, pale buff or cream coloured powder with slightly earthy test. It is insoluble in water but swells to approximately twelve times its volume when water is added. It is insoluble in organic solvents in which it does not swell.

Identification Tests : Identification tests are performed mainly on the basis of the presence of aluminium ion.

Fuse the sample (1 g) with anhydrous sodium carbonate (2 g). Warm the residue with distilled water (10 ml). Filter and wash the filtrate with water (5 ml). Combine the filtrate and washings. The residue is tested for the presence of aluminium and filtrate for silica.

Tests for Aluminium : Dissolve the residue in dilute hydrochloric acid (10 ml) and perform the following tests.

(1) Take the above solution (2 ml), add thioacetamide reagent (0.5 ml), no precipitate is formed. Add dropwise 2 N sodium hydroxide solution, a gelatinous white precipitate of aluminium hydroxide is obtained.

$$AlCl_3 + 3NaOH \longrightarrow Al(OH)_3 \downarrow + 3NaCl$$

The precipitate is redissolved on addition of excess of sodium hydroxide solution due to formation of tetrahydroxy aluminate but re-appears on addition of ammonium chloride solution.

$$Al(OH)_3 + NaOH \longrightarrow [Al(OH)_4]^- Na^+$$

Sodium tetrahydroxy aluminate solution.

$$[Al(OH)_4]^- Na^+ + NH_4Cl \longrightarrow Al(OH)_3 + NH_3 + NaCl + H_2O.$$

(2) To the above solution (2 ml), add few drops of freshly prepared 0.05% w/v solution of quinalizarin in 1% w/v solution of sodium hydroxide, boil, cool and acidify with excess of acetic acid; a reddish-violet colour is produced.

Aluminium is precipitated into aluminium hydroxide in the presence of the dye, quinalizarin. The hydroxide forms a coloured lake with the dye. The aluminium complex is reddish violet in acetric acid solution (see chapter 5).

Test for Silica :

(3) To the above filtrate and washings, add dilute hydrochloric acid (3 ml), a gelatinous precipitate of metasilicic acid, H_2SiO_3, is formed.

Calcium Gluconate, $C_{12}H_{22}CaO_{14}$, H_2O

It is used as an electrolyte replenisher. It is an odourless, tasteless, white crystalline powder. Calcium gluconate is slightly soluble in water, freely soluble in boiling water and insoluble in alcohol.

Identification Tests : Identification tests are performed on the basis of presence of calcium and D-gluconic acid.

Tests for Gluconic Acid

(1) To a solution of 3% w/v calcium gluconate (1 ml), add few drops of ferric chloride solution, a yellow colour appears. Gluconic acid is an α-hydroxy acid. It reacts with ferric chloride to form a yellow coloured complex.

(2) To the sample (0.75 g) in warm water (7.5 ml), add glacial acetic acid (1 ml) and freshly distilled phenylhydrazine (1.5 ml). Heat the mixture on a water bath for half an hour and allow to cool. Scratch the inner surface of the tube with a glass rod until crystals of gluconic acid phenylhydrazine begin to form. Keep the test tube for 10 minutes, filter, dissolve the precipitate in hot water (10 ml), add a small amount of decolourizing charcoal and filter. Allow to cool and scratch the test tube to recover the white crystals which melt at about 200° with decomposition.

Phenylhydrazine forms gluconic acid phenylhydrazide with gluconic acid which is purified by boiling with charcoal and identified on the basis of melting point determination.

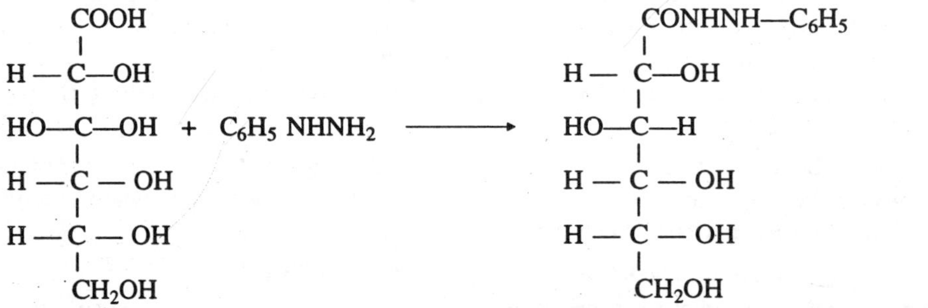

Gluconic Acid — Gluconic Acid Phenylhydrazide

Test for Calcium Ion :

(3) To a little quantity of calcium gluconate, add few drops of a solution of ammonium oxalate. A white precipitate is obtained which is slightly soluble in dilute acetic acid but soluble in hydrochloric acid

$$Ca^{++} \xrightarrow{\text{Ammonium oxalate solution}} \underset{\substack{\text{Calcium oxilate} \\ \text{(White ppt)}}}{Ca(COO)_2}$$

(4) Dissolve the calcium gluconate solution (20 ml) in minimum quantity of dilute hydrochloric acid and neutralize with dilute sodium hydroxide solution. Add ammonium carbonate solution (5 ml), a white precipitate is formed which after boiling and cooling the mixture is only sparingly soluble in ammonium chloride solution.

Calcium ion reacts with ammonium carbonate to form a white precipitate of calcium carbonate.

$$Ca^{++} \xrightarrow{\text{Ammonium carbonate}} \underset{\text{White precipitate}}{CaCO_3}$$

(5) Dissolve the calcium gluconate solution (20 ml) in glacial acetic acid (1 ml). Add potassium ferrocyanide (0.5 ml), the solution remains clear. Add ammonium chloride (50 ml), a white precipitate, due to formation of ammonium calcium ferrocyanide, $(NH_4)_2\ Ca\ [Fe\ (CN)_6]$, is produced.

Ferrous Gluconate:

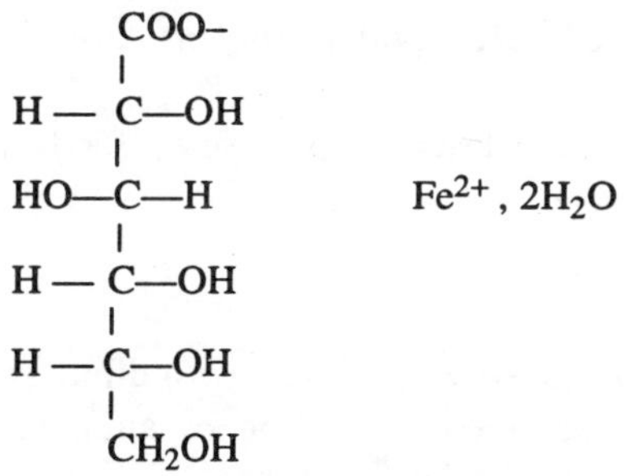

Ferrous gluconate is haematinic in action. It is yellowish-grey or pale greenish yellow fine powder. Its odour is slightly resembles with burnt sugars. Ferrous gluconate is soluble in water but insoluble in alcohol

Indentification Tests : Identification tests are based on reaction of ferrous ion and D-gluconic acid.

Tests for D-Gluconic Acid:

(1) Carry out the same tests as in case of calcium gluconate for gluconic acid.

Tests for Ferrous Ion:

A solution (1 in 20) gives the reactions of ferrous salt.

(1) Take solution of ferrous gluconate (2 ml), add dilute sulphuric acid (2 ml) and 0.1% w/v solution of 1, 10-phenanthroline (1 ml). An intense red colour is produced; the colour is discharged by addition of slight excess of 0.1N ceric ammonium sulphate.

Ferrous ion forms red coloured complx with 1,10-phenanthroline (see chapter 3). The colour disappears on addition of ceric ammonium sulphate due to oxidation of ferrous ion into ferric ion.

(2) Take solution of ferrous gluconate (1 ml), add potassium ferricyanide solution (1 ml), a dark blue precipitate is formed which is insoluble in dilute hydrochloric acid and is decomposed by sodium hydroxide solution. Ferricyanide oxidizes ferrous into ferric,

themselves reduces into ferrocyanide $[Fe(CN)_6]^{4-}$.

$$Fe^{2+} + [Fe(CN)_6]^{3-} \longrightarrow Fe^{+++} + [Fe(CN)_6]^{2-}$$

Ferrocyanide ion reacts with ferric ions to form dark blue colour due to formation of ferriferricyanide

$$4Fe^{+++} + 3[Fe(CN)]^{4-} \longrightarrow Fe_4\,[Fe\,(CN_6]_3.$$

(3) Take solution of ferrous gluconate (1 ml), add potassium ferrocyanide solution (1 ml), a white precipitate is formed due to formation of potassium ferroferrocyanide which rapidly becomes blue in colour in presence of oxygen.

$$Fe^{++} + 2K^{++} + [Fe(CH)_6]^{4-} \longrightarrow K_2\,Fe[Fe(CN)_6]\downarrow$$

$$4K_2Fe[Fe(CN)_6] + 4H^+ + O_2 \longrightarrow 4KFe[Fe(CN)_6] + 4K^+ + 2H_2O$$

The precipitate is insoluble in dilute hydrochloric acid solution.

Ferric Ammonium Citrate

It is haematinic, used in iron deficiency. It occurs as thin, transparent, dark red scales or granules or a brownish-red granular powder; odourless with astringent taste. It is very soluble in water but insoluble in alcohol.

Identification Tests : Identification tests are performed for ferric ion, ammonium ion and citrate ion.

Test for Ammonium Ion:

1. Heat ferric ammonium citrate solution (2 ml) with dilute solution of sodium hydroxide (1 ml). Ammonia gas is evolved. Evolution of ammonia indicates the presence of ammonium ion.

Test for Citrates:

Take the above solution, add calcium chloride solution (1 ml) and boil. A white precipitate of calcium citrate is formed. This white precipitate is soluble in acetic acid solution.

$$\begin{array}{lcll} CH_2COOH & & & CH_2 - COOCa \\ | & & & | \\ C(OH)\,COOH & + & CaCl_2 \longrightarrow & C\,(OH)\,COOCa \\ | & & & | \\ CH_2COOH & & & CH_2-COOCa \\ \text{Citric Acid} & & & \text{Calcium Citrate} \end{array}$$

1. To the above solution (5 ml), add sulphuric acid (0.5 ml), potassium permanganate solution (3 ml) and warm until the colour of the permanganate is discharged. Add 10% w/v solution of sodium nitroprusside (0.5 ml) in 2N sulphuric acid and sulphamic acid (4 g). Make alkaline with strong ammonia solution, added dropwise until all the sulphamic acid has dissolved. Add more of strong ammonia solution, a violet colour is produced which changes into violet-blue colour.
   Citrate decolourizes acidified potassium permanganate due to oxidation into carbon monoxide and acetone dicarboxylic acid.

$$\text{Citrate} \xrightarrow{KMnO_4} CO + \underset{\text{Acetone diacarboxylic acid}}{HOOC\,CH_2\,\overset{\overset{O}{\|}}{C}\,CH_2\,COOH} \longrightarrow CH_3\overset{\overset{O}{\|}}{C}CH_3 + CO_2$$

Acetone diacarboxylic acid ↓ Sodium nitroprusside

$$\text{Violet colour} \xrightarrow{\text{Sulphamic acid}} \text{Violet-blue colour}$$

Acetone dicarboxylic acid is converted into acetone. It also reacts with sodium nitroprusside, $Na_2\,[Fe\,(CN)_5\,NO]\,2H_2O$, in the presence of sulphamic acid, $NH_2\,SO_3H$, gives a violet colour which changes into violet-blue colour.

Tests for Ferric Salt :

Gently ignite the sample in a China dish. Dissolve the residue in hydrochloric acid. Carry out the following tests with the solution :

2. To the solution (1 ml), add 5% w/v solution of potassium ferrocyanide (1 ml). An intense blue precipitate is formed due to formation of ferriferrocyanide, $Fe_4\,[Fe\,(CN)_6]_3$.

$$Fe^{+++} \xrightarrow{HCl} FeCl_2$$

$$4FeCl_3 + \underset{\text{Potassium ferrocyanide}}{3K_4\,[Fe\,(CN)_6]} \longrightarrow \underset{\text{Ferriferrocyanide}}{Fe_4\,[Fe\,(CN)_6]} + 12\ KCl$$

3. To the above solution (4 ml), add ammonium thiocyanate solution (1 ml). Red colour is produced due to formation of ferric thiocyanate.

$$FeCl_3 + NH_4\,SCN \longrightarrow \underset{\text{Ferric thiocyanate}}{Fe\,(SCN)_3} + 3NH_4\,Cl\ Fe$$

Divide this solution into two portions. To one portion add ether (5 ml), shake and allow to stand. The ether layer becomes pink due to solubility of ferric thiocyanate in ether. To another portion add 0.2M mercuric chloride (3 ml). The red colour disappears due to formation of non-dissociated mercuric thiocyanate $Hg(SCN)_2$.

$$2Fe\,(SCN)_3 + 3HgCl_2 \longrightarrow \underset{\text{Mercuric thiocynate}}{3Hg\,(SCN)_2} + 2Fe\,Cl_3$$

4. To the above solution (3 ml), add acetic acid followed by addition of 0.2% w/v solution of 8-hydroxy 7-iodoquinoline-5-sulphonic acid (2 ml). A stable green colour is produced. The reagent 8-hydroxy 7-iodiquinoline-5-sulphonic acid, also called ferron reagent, forms green coloured complex in acidic medium (see chapter 5)

Ferrous Sulphate, $Fe\,SO_4 . 7H_2O$

It is a Haematinic compound, available as transparent, green crystals or as a pale bluish green, crystalline powder. It is efflorescent in dry air and on exposure to moist air, the crystals rapidly oxidize and become coated with brownish yellow basic ferrous sulphate.

It is soluble in water but insoluble in alcohol.

Identification Tests : Identification tests are performed for the ferrous salts and sulphates

Tests for Ferrous Salts :

Carry out the same tests for ferrous salts as in ferrous gluconate.

Tests for Sulphate :

(1) Take the solution of ferrous sulphate (1 g in 20 ml) (5 ml) in a test tube, add dilute

hydrochloric acid (1 ml) and barium chloride solution (1 ml), a white precipitate or turbidity appears due to formation of barium sulphate.

$$FeSO_4 + BaCl_2 \longrightarrow \underset{\text{Barium sulphate.}}{BaSO_4} + FeCl_2$$

(2) Add lead acetate solution (2 ml) to ferrous sulphate solution (5 ml); a white precipitate of lead sulphate is formed.

Hydrogen Peroxide, H_2O_2

It is an antiseptic and topical anti-infective agent. It occurs as a colourless, odourless liquid with slightly acidic taste. It contains not less than 5% w/v and not more than 7% w/v of H_2O_2 corresponding to about 20 times its volume of available oxygen.

Identification Tests :

(1) Add dilute sodium hydroxide solution (1 ml) and heat. Oxygen is evolved due to decomposition.

$$2H_2O_2 \longrightarrow 2H_2O + O_2$$

(2) One drop of hydrogen peroxide solution is acidifed with (2 ml) dilute sulphuric acid and shaked well. Add one drop of potassium chromate solution and solvent ether (2 ml), the ethereal layer is coloured blue due to formation of chromium pentoxide, CrO_5, which is more soluble in diethyl ether.

$$K_2CrO_4 + H_2SO_4 + 2H_2O_2 \longrightarrow CrO_5 + K_2SO_4 + 3H_2O.$$

Iodine, I_2

Iodine is a topical anti-infective agent. It occurs as heavy, bluish-black, rhombic prism or plates with a metallic lustre and characteristic odour. It is volatile at room temperature. It is slightly soluble in water, soluble in alcohol, freely soluble in carbon disulphide, chloroform, solvent ether, carbon tetrachloride and concentrated aqueous solution of iodides.

Identification Tests : (1) On gentle heating, it gives violet coloured vapours which condense forming a bluish-black crystalline sublimate.

(2) Dissolve few crystals of iodine in potassium iodide solution and add few drops of starch mucilage. A deep blue colour is produced which disappears on boiling but re-appears on cooling.

Magnesium Sulphate, $MgSO_4.7H_2O$

Synonym : Epsom Salts:

It occurs as odourless, colourless crystals with cool, saline and bitter taste. It effloresces in warm dry air. Its one part is soluble in 1 part of water but slightly soluble in alcohol and dissolves slowly in 1 part of glycerin.

Identification Tests : It gives reactions characteristic of magnesium and sulphate.

Tests for Magnesium : Prepare a solution (1 in 20) of the given sample and perform the following tests.

(1) To the above solution (2 ml), add dilute ammonia solution (1 ml). A white precipitate of magnesium hydroxide is formed.

$$MgSO_4 + 2NH_4OH \longrightarrow Mg(OH)_2\downarrow + (NH_4)_2SO_4$$

The precipitate dissolves on addition of 2 M ammonium chloride solution (1 ml). To this solution, add 0.025 M disodium hydrogen phosphate solution (1 ml) to obtain white precipitate of magnesium ammonium phosphate, Mg (NH_4) PO_4.

$$Mg^{2+} + NH_3 + HPO_4^{2-} \longrightarrow \underset{\text{Magnesium ammonium phosphate}}{Mg(NH_4)PO_4}$$

Test for Sulphate : Carry out the same test as in barium sulphate.

Mercuric Oxide Yellow , HgO

It contains not less than 99% of HgO, calculated with reference to the substance, and dried at 105° for one hour.

It is an orange yellow, heavy, amorphous powder. It is odourless, stable is air but becomes discoloured on exposure to light. It is antibacterial in action.

Identification tests

(1) On heating gently, it produces red colour but on strong heating, it decomposes into oxygen and mercury.

(2) Acidic solution of mercuric oxide gives white precipitate with sodium hydroxide solution.

(3) Potassium iodide solution is added to a neutral solution. Scarlet precipitate is produced due to formation of Hg_2I_2 which is soluble in excess of potassium iodide solution.

Potassium Permanganate, $KMnO_4$

It is a topical anti-infective agent. It occurs as dark purple, prismatic crystals with metallic lustre. It is odourless with sweet astringent taste. Potassium permanganate is soluble in water and freely soluble in boiling water.

Identification Tests : It gives reactions characteristic of permanganate and potassium ions.

Test for Permanganate : To the aqueous potassium permanganate solution (2 ml), add dilute sulphuric acid (1 ml) and warm to 70°. Add hydrogen peroxide solution. Permanganate solution is decolourized, due to oxidation of hydrogen peroxide and conversion of permanganate ion into colourless manganese ions.

$$2KMnO_4 + 5H_2O_2 + 3H_2SO_4 \longrightarrow 5O_2 \uparrow + 2MnSO_4 + K_2SO_4 + 8H_2O$$

Tests for Potassium : The compound is heated to redness, it decrepitates, evolves oxygen and leaves a black residue which forms potassium hydroxide on addition of few ml of water. Neutralize the solution with dilute hydrochloric acid solution and perform the following tests with the resulting solution.

(1) Take the above solution (1 ml), add dilute acetic acid (1 ml) and freshly prepared 10% w/v solution of sodium cobaltinitrite (1 ml). A yellow or orange precipitate of potassium cobaltinitrite, $K_3 [Co (NO_2)_6]$, is formed.

$$CH_3COOK + Na_3 [Co(NO_2)_6] \longrightarrow \underset{\text{Potassium cobaltinitrite}}{K_3 [Co (NO_2)_6]} + 3CH_3 COONa$$

(2) Take the above solution (2 ml), add sodium carbonate solution (1 ml) and heat. No precipitation appears. Add sodium sulphate solution (0.5 ml); no precipitate occurs. Cool in ice bath. Add 15% w/v solution of tartaric acid (2 ml), a white precipitate is formed due to formation of potassium hydrogen tartarate.

$$CH_3COOK + \begin{array}{l} CH(OH)COOH \\ | \\ CH(OH)COOH \end{array} \longrightarrow \begin{array}{l} CH(OH)COOK \\ | \\ CH(OH)COOH \end{array} + CH_3COOH$$

Tartaric acid — Potassium hydrogen tartrate

Potassium Iodide, KI

Potassium iodide is used as an antifungal, expectorant and source of iodine. It occurs as colourless crystals or white powder. It is odourless with saline and slightly bitter taste. Potassium permanganate is soluble in water, glycerin and alcohol.

Identification Tests : It gives reactions characteristic of potassium and iodides.

Test for Potassium : Carry out the same test as for potassium permanganate.

Tests for Iodides

(1) Take potassium iodide solution (2 ml), acidify with dilute nitric acid, add silver nitrate solution (0.5 ml) and shake. A pale yellow precipitate appears due to formation of silver iodide.

$$KI + AgNO_3 \xrightarrow{HNO_3} \underset{\substack{\text{Silver iodide} \\ \text{(Yellow ppt)}}}{AgI} + KNO_3$$

The precipitate is insoluble in ammonia solution.

(2) Take a solution of potassium iodide (2 ml), add 2N sulphuric acid (0.5 ml), potassium dichromate solution (0.15 ml), water (2 ml), and chloroform (2 ml). Shake for few seconds and allow to stand. The chloroform layer becomes violet or violet-red in colour. Potassium iodide is oxidized by potassium dichromate and liberates iodine which is more soluble in chloroform and so violet colour is produced.

$$6I^- + 14H^+ + Cr_2O_7^{\ 2-} \longrightarrow 2Cr^{3+} + 7H_2O + 3I_2$$

(3) Take a solution containing equivalent of about 5 mg of iodide ion and add mercuric chloride solution (0.5 ml). A dark red precipitate is formed which is slightly soluble in an excess of this reagent and very soluble in an excess of potassium iodide solution forming potassium mercuri iodide.

$$2I^- + HgCl_2 \longrightarrow HgI_2 + 2Cl^-$$

$$HgI_2 + 2I^- \longrightarrow \underset{\text{complex salt}}{[HgI_4]^{2-}}$$

Sodium benzoate, C_6H_5COONa.

Sodium benzoate is a pharmaceutical aid, most commonly used as antifungal preservative. It is white, amorphous, granular or crystalline powder. It is odourless or with faint odour, and its taste is unpleasant, sweetish and saline. It is freely soluble in water and slightly soluble in alcohol.

Identification Tests : Sodium benzoate gives reactions for benzoic acid and for sodium ions.

Tests for Benzoic Acid:

(1) To a 10% w/v solution, add ferric chloride solution. A buff coloured precipitate is produced due to formation of basic ferric benzoate. The precipitate is soluble in dilute

hydrochloric acid.

$$3C_6H_5\,COONa + 2FeCl_3 + 3H_2O \longrightarrow \underset{\text{Ferric benzoate}}{(C_6H_5COO)_3Fe.Fe(OH)_3} + 3NaCl + 3HCl$$

(2) Dissolve the substance (0.5 g) in water (5 ml). Add hydrochloric acid (0.5 ml). A precipitate of benzoic acid appears which is filtered, washed and dried; its melting point should be 120°.

$$C_6H_5COONa + HCl \longrightarrow \underset{\text{Benzoic acid}}{C_6H_5COOH} + NaCl$$

Tests for Sodium : Prepare a solution (1 in 20) of the substance and carry out the following tests:

1. Take the above solution (2 ml), add 15% w/v solution of potassium carbonate (2 ml) and heat to boiling; no precipitate forms. Add freshly prepared potassium antimonate solution (4 ml) and heat to boiling. Cool in an ice bath. Rub, if necessary, the inside layer of the test tube with a glass rod. A dense white precipitate is formed due to formation of sodium antimonate.

$$\underset{\text{Potassium antimonate}}{KSbO_3} + Na^+ \longrightarrow \underset{\text{Sodium antimonate}}{NaSbO_3} \downarrow + K^+$$

(2) Acidify the above solution (1 ml) with acetic acid. Add an excess of magnesium uranyl acetate solution. A yellow crystalline precipitate is formed.
Magnesium uranyl acetate solution is of uranyl acetate, $UO_2\,(CH_3\,COO)_2$, and magnesium acetate, $Mg\,(CH_3COO)_2$, in dilute acetic acid. Sodium ions on reaction with this reagent form white precipitate of sodium magnesium uranyl acetate.

$$Na^+ + Mg^{++} + 3UO_2^- + 9CH_3COO^- \longrightarrow \underset{\text{Sodium magnesium uranyl acetate.}}{NaMg(UO_2)_3(CH_3COO)_9}$$

Sodium Bicarbonate, $NaHCO_3$

It is used as an electrolyte replenisher and systemic alkalinizer. Sodium bicarbonate is a white crystalline powder. It is odourless with saline taste. Sodium bicarbonate is soluble in water but insoluble in alcohol.

Identification Tests : It gives reactions of sodium and bicarbonates.

Tests for Sodium :

Carry out the same tests as in sodium benzoate.

Tests for Bicarbonate:

(1) Boil the solution; carbon dioxide gas is liberated.

$$2NaHCO_3\,. \longrightarrow Na_2\,CO_3 + H_2O + CO_2 \uparrow$$

(2) To the sodium bicarbonate solution (1 ml), add solution of magnesium sulphate (1 ml); no precipitate is formed but white precipitate is obtained on boiling the solution, due to formation of magnesium carbonate.

$$Mg^{++} + 2H\,CO_3^- \longrightarrow \underset{\text{Magnesium carbonate}}{Mg\,CO_3} + H_2O + CO_2$$

(3) Add 2N acetic acid solution (2 ml) to a solution of the substance (0.1 g in 2 ml of water). Close the tube immediately using a stopper filted with a glass tube bent at two right angles. Heat gently and pass the generated carbon dioxide gas into barium hydroxide solution (5 ml); a white precipitate of barium carbonate appears which is soluble in dilute hydrochloric acid.

$$NaHCO_3 + CH_3COOH \longrightarrow CH_3COONa + H_2O + CO_2 \uparrow$$

$$CO_2 + Ba(OH)_2 \longrightarrow \underset{\text{Barium carbonate (White ppt)}}{BaCO_3} + H_2O$$

$$BaCO_3 + 2HCl \longrightarrow BaCl_2 + CO_2 + H_2O.$$

Sodium Chloride, NaCl.

Sodium chloride is used as a pharmaceutical aid. It is an odourless, colourless or white crystalline powder with saline taste. It is soluble in water, glycerin and slightly soluble in alcohol.

Identification Tests : It is identified on the basis of presence of sodium ion and chloride ion. Carry out the same tests for sodium as in sodium benzoate and for chloride as in ammonium chloride.

Sodium Thiosulphate, $Na_2S_2O_3 . 5H_2O$

It is used as antidote to cyanide poisoning. It occurs as an odourless, colourless crystalline mass or coarsely crystalline powder with saline taste. It is deliquescent in moist air and effloresces in dry air at temperature above 30°.

Identification Tests : It gives characteristic reactions of sodium ion and thiosulphate. It is also identified on the basis of its reducing properties.

(1) To a 10% w/v solution, add few drops of iodine solution; the colour is discharged. It is an oxidation-reduction reaction. Iodine is an oxidizing agent and so reduced into iodide, which is colourless.

$$Na_2S_2O_3 + I_2 \longrightarrow 2NaI + \underset{\text{Sodium tetrathionate}}{Na_2S_4O_6}$$

(2) Solution of thiosulphate decolourizes bromine solution; the decolourized solution give the reactions of sulphate.

(3) Dissolve the substance (0.1 g) in water (5 ml), add dilute hydrochloric acid (2 ml). A white precipitate, which soon turns yellow due to separation of sulphur, recognized by its characteristic odour.

$$Na_2S_2O_3 + 2HCl \longrightarrow S \downarrow + SO_2 \uparrow + H_2O + 2NaCl$$

(4) Dissolve the substance (0.1 g) in water (5 ml) and add ferric chloride solution (2 ml). A deep violet colour is produced which quickly disappears.

Zinc Sulphate, $ZnSO_4 . 7H_2O$

Zinc sulphate contains not less than 99% and not more than 104% of $ZnSO_4 . 7H_2O$.

It occurs as colourless, odourless, transparent crystals or white, crystalline powder. It is efforescent in nature. It is highly soluble in water but practically insoluble in 95% alcohol. It is used as astringent.

Identification Tests : Dissolve 2.5 g in sufficient amount of carbon dioxide free water to produce 50 ml. This solution gives the reactions of zinc salt and sulphate.

Tests for Zinc Salt

(1) Take the above solution (5 ml), add sodium hydroxide solution (10.2 ml); white precipitate is produced. Add further sodium hydroxide solution (2 ml), the precipitate dissolves. Add ammonium chloride solution (10 ml), the solution remains clear. Add sodium sulphide solution (0.1 ml), a flocculent white precipitate is produced.

(2) Acidify the above solution (5 ml) with dilute sulphuric acid, add one drop of 0.1% w/v cupric sulphate solution and ammonium mercurithiocyanate solution (2 ml); a violet precipitate is formed.

(3) To the above solution (5 ml), add potassium ferrocyanide solution (2 ml), a white precipitate, insoluble in dilute hydrochloric acid, is produced.

Test for sulphate : Carry out the same tests as for barium sulphate.

Zinc Oxide, ZnO

Zinc oxide contains not less than 99% and not more than 100.5% of ZnO, calculated with reference to ignited substance.

It is available as soft, white or faintly yellowish white amorphous powder, free from grittiness. It gradually absorbs carbon dioxide from the air. It is used as mild astringent and topical protective.

Identification Tests

(1) It becomes yellow when strongly heated; the yellow colour diasppears on cooling.

(2) Dissolve zinc oxide (0.1 g) in 2 M hydrochloric acid solution (1.5 ml) and add sufficient water to make up the 5 ml. This solution gives the characteristic reactions of zinc salt as in zinc sulphate.

7

Limit Tests

Every pharmaceutical substance contains some impurities varying in proportion. Indian Pharmacopoeia has fixed a limit of these impurities. To check the limit, some official tests, called limit tests, are carried out.

Limit tests involve the comparison of opalescence, turbidity or colour with fixed standards. The extent of opalescence, turbidity and colour is affected by the presence of other impurities present in the substance, variation in time and method of performance of the tests. Generally an aqueous solution of substance is prepared. Sometimes a solution of the substance is prepared by dissolving in an acid or, if the solution is alkaline, it is neutralized with nitric acid or hydrochloric acid.

Limit Test for Chloride

It involves the reaction of silver nitrate with soluble chlorides to form the precipitate of silver chloride which is insoluble in dilute nitric acid. The extent of precipitate depends upon the amount of silver chloride formed or amount of chloride ions present in the substance. The opalescence produced is compared with a standard oplescence obtained from standard solution containing fixed amount of chloride under the same experimental conditions.

$$NaCl + AgNO_3 \xrightarrow{\text{dil } HNO_3} \underset{\text{White ppt}}{AgCl \downarrow} + NaNO_3$$

Method :

Standard Opalescence
Place 0.05845% w/v solution of sodium chloride (1 ml) and dilute nitric acid (10 ml) in a Nesselar cylinder. Dilute to 50 ml with water and add silver nitrate solution (1 ml). Stir immediately with glass rod and allow to stand and five minutes.

Test Opalescence
Dissolve the specified quantity of the substance in water and transfer to a Nessler cylinder. Add dilute nitric acid solution (10 ml) except when it is used in the preparation of the solution. Stir immediately with a glass rod and allow to stand for 5 minutes.

Observe the opalescence in both the solutions (views transversely). The opalescence produced should not be *greater than the standard opalescence.*

Limit Test for Sulphate

Limit test for sulphate is based on the reaction between barium chloride and soluble sulphate in the presence of dilute hydrochloric acid. The turbidity formed in the test solution is compared with the standard turbidity obtained by the fixed quantity of the sulphate under the same experimental conditions.

$$BaCl_2 + Na_2SO_4 \longrightarrow \underset{\text{White precipitate.}}{BaSO_4} + 2NaCl$$

Method

Standard Opalescence

Place a 0.1089% w/v solution of potassium sulphate (1 ml) and dilute hydrochloric acid (2 ml) in a Nessler cylinder, dilute to 45 ml of water, add barium sulphate reagent (5 ml), stir immediately with a glass rod and allow to stand for five minutes.

Test Solution Opalescence

Dissolve the specified quantity of the substance in water, or prepare a solution as directed in the text, transfer to a Nesseler cylinder and add dilute hydrochloric acid (2 ml) except where hydrochloric acid is used in preparation of the solution. Dilute to 45 ml with water, add barium sulphate reagent (5 ml), stir immediately with a glass rod and allow to stand for five minutes.

The opalescence produced by the test solution should not be greater than standard opalescence when viewed transversely.

Barium Sulphate Reagents

Mix solution (15 ml) 0.5 M barium chloride, water (55 ml) and sulphate free alcohol (20 ml). Add 0.181% w/v potassium sulphate solution (5 ml), dilute to 100 ml with water and mix. Barium sulphate reagent must be freshly prepared.

0.5 M Barium Chloride solution : It contain barium chloride, $BaCl_2 \cdot 2H_2O$ (122.18 g), dissolved in water (1000 ml).

Limit Test for Iron

The limit test for iron depends on the reaction of iron in ammonical solution in the presence of citric acid with thioglycollic acid to obtain a pale pink to deep reddish purple colour. Citric acid forms a complex with iron which is not precipitated by ammonia. The colour is obtained due to formation of ferrous salt, $Fe(SCH_2COO)_2$, which disappears in air due to oxidation.

$$\underset{\text{Thioglycollic acid}}{2HSCH_2COOH} + \text{Ferrous or Ferric ion} \longrightarrow \underset{\text{Ferrous thioglycollate}}{Fe(HSCH_2COO)_2} + 2H^+$$

The colour produced in the test solution is compared from a known amount of iron under the same experimental conditions.

Method

Standard Colour

Dilute standard iron solution (2 ml) with water (40 ml) in a Nesseler cylinder. Add 20% w/v solution of iron free citric acid (2 ml) and thioglycollic acid (0.1 ml), mix, make alkaline with iron free ammonia solution, dilute to 50 ml with water and allow to stand for five minutes.

Test Solution Colour

Dissolve the specified quantity of the substance being examined in water (40 ml) or use of this solution (10 ml) prescribed in the monograph. Add 20% w/v solution of iron free citric acid (2 ml) and thioglycollic acid (0.1 ml), mix, make alkaline with iron free ammonia solution, dilute to 50 ml with water and allow to stand for five minutes.

Standard Iron Solution : Weight accurately ferric ammonium sulphate (0.1726 g) and dissolve in 0.1N H_2SO_4 solution (10 ml) and sufficient water to produce 1000 ml. Each ml of this solution contains 0.02 mg of Fe.

Limit Test for Heavy Metals.

The test for heavy metals is designed to determine the content of metallic impurities that are coloured by sulphide ion, under the specified conditions. The limit for heavy metals is indicated in the individual monographs in terms of part of lead per million parts of the substance (by weight) as determined by visual comparison of the colour produced by the substance with that of the control prepared from standard lead solution.

The amount of heavy metals is determined by one of the following methods and as directed in the individual monograph:

Method A is used for substances that yield clear, colourless solutions under the specified test condition. Method B is used for substances that do not yield clear, colourless solutions under the test conditions specified for Method A, or for substances which, by virtue of their complex nature, interfere with the precipitation of metals by sulphide ion. Method C is used for substances that yield clear, colourless solutions with sodium hydroxide solution.

Method A

Standard Colour

Into a 50 ml Nessler cylinder. standard lead solution (2 ml) is pipetted and diluted with water to 25 ml, adjusted with dilute acetic acid Sp. or dilute ammonia solution Sp. to a pH between 3.0 and 4.0, dilute with water to about 35 ml, and mixed. Add freshly prepared hydrogen sulphide solution (10 ml), mix, dilute with water to 50 ml, allow to stand for five minutes and view downwards over a white surface.

Test Colour

Into a 50 ml Nessler cylinder, the test solution (25 ml) is prepared, adjusted with dilute acetic acid Sp. or dilute ammonia solution Sp. to a pH between 3.0 and 4.0, diluted with water to about 35 ml and mixed. Add freshly prepared hydrogen sulphide solution (10 ml), mix, dilute with water to 50 ml, allow to stand for five minutes and view downwards over a white surface.

The colour produced in the test solution should not be darker than that produced in the standard solution.

Method B

Standard Colour

Proceed as directed under Method A.

Test Colour

In a suitable crucible, the quantity of the substance is weighed, sufficient sulphuric acid Sp. added to wet the sample, and ignited carefully at a low temperature until thoroughly charred. To the charred mass, nitric acid Sp. (2 ml) and five drops of sulphuric acid Sp. are added: heated cautiously until white fumes are no longer evolved, ignited preferably in a muffle furnace at 500° to 600°, until the carbon is completely burnt off. It is cooled, hydrochloric acid Sp. (4 ml) is added, covered, digested on a water-bath for 15 minutes, uncovered and slowly evaporated to dryness on a water-bath. The residue is moistened with one drop of hydrochloric acid Sp., followed by addition of hot water (10 ml) and digested for two minutes. Ammonia solution Sp. is added dropwise, until the solution is just alkaline to litmus paper, diluted with water to 25 ml and adjusted with dilute acetic acid Sp., to a pH between 3.0 and 4.0. It is filtered, if necessary, the crucible rinsed and filtered with water (10 ml). The filtrate and washings are combined in a 50 ml Nessler cylinder, diluted with water to about 35 ml, and mixed. Add freshly prepared hydrogen sulphide solution (10 ml), mix, dilute with water to 50 ml, allow to stand for five minutes and view downwards over a white surface.

The colour produced in the test solution should not be darker than the colour of the standard solution.

Method C

Standard Colour

Into a 50 ml Nessler cylinder, standard lead solution (2 ml) is pipetted, dilute sodium hydroxide solution (5 ml) added, diluted with water to 50 ml and mixed. Add 5 drops of solution sulphide solution, mix, allow to stand for 5 minutes and view downwards over a white surface.

Test Colour

Into a 50 ml Nessler cylinder, the test solution (25 ml) prepared are placed, the specified quantity dissolved in a mixture of water (20 ml) and dilute sodium hydroxide solution (5 ml). It is diluted to 50 ml with water and mixed. Add 5 drops of sodium sulphide solution, mix, allow to stand for 5 minutes and view downwards over a white surface.

The colour produced in the test solution should not be darker than the colour of the standard solution.

Standard Lead Solution : On the day of use, dilute lead nitrate stock solution (10 ml) with water to 100 ml. Each ml of standard lead solution contains the equivalent of 10 μg of lead.

Lead Nitrate Stock Solution : Dissolve lead nitrate (0.1598 g) in water (100 ml) to which has been added nitric acid (1 ml), then dilute with water to 1000.0 ml.

This solution must be prepared and stored in a polyethylene or glass container free from soluble lead salt.

Limit Test for Lead

Lead is a toxic substance present in pharmaceutical preparations. The main sources of this impurity are sulphuric acid and the lead apparatus. The I.P. and U.S.P. method is based on the reaction between lead and dithizone (diphenylthiocarbazone). In chloroform solution, dithizone extracts lead from an alkaline aqueous solution as lead dithizonate which has red colour in chloroform solution. Since dithizone itself imparts a green colour in chloroform, the resultant colour of dithizone and lead dithizone is violet. The colour produced by a given amount of the sample is compared with that produced by a known volume of a standard solution of lead. If the colour is intense than that produced by the standard, it contains lead in excess of prescribed limit. For the test, the lead present as impurity is separated by extracting an alkaline solution of the substance with dithizone extraction solution which removes all the lead in the form of its complex in chloroform layer.

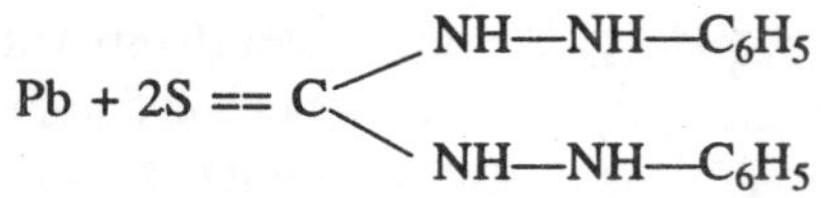

Diphenyl Thiocarbazone (Dithizone)

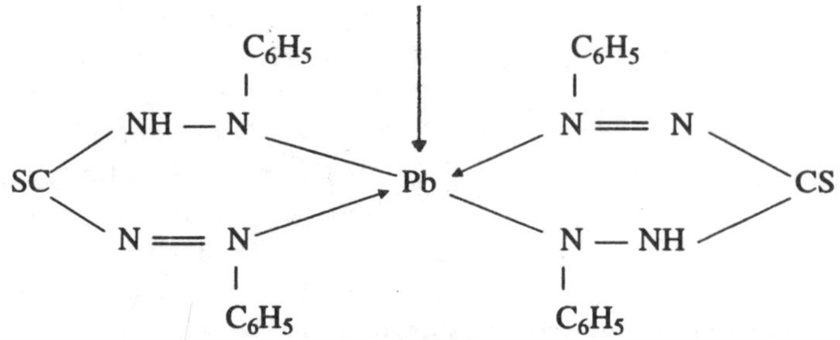

Lead dithizonate

Method

The volume of the prepared sample in a separator is transferred and unless otherwise directed in monograph, ammonium citrate solution Sp. (6 ml), and hydroxylamine hydrochloride solution Sp. (2 ml) are added (For the determination of lead in iron salts use ammonium citrate solution Sp. (10 ml)). Two drops of phenol red solution are added and the solution is made just alkaline (red in colour) by the addition of strong ammonia solution. The solution is cooled, if necessary, and potassium cyanide solution Sp. (2 ml) is added. Immediately the solution is extracted with several quantities, each of 5 ml, of dithizone extraction solution, draining off each extract into another separating funnel, until the dithizone extraction solution retains its green colour. The combined dithizone solutions are shaken for 30 seconds with 1 per cent w/v solution of nitric acid (30 ml) and the chloroform layer discarded. To the acid solution, standard dithizone solution (5 ml) and ammonia-cyanide solution Sp. (5 ml) are added and shaken for 30 seconds; the colour of the chloroform layer is of no deeper shade of violet than that of a control made with a volume of dilute standard lead solution equivalent to the amount of lead permitted in the sample under examination.

All reagents used for the test should have as low a content of lead as practicable. All reagent solutions should be stored in containers of borosilicate glass. Glassware should be rinsed thoroughly with warm dilute nitric acid, followed by water.

Standard Dithizone Solution : Dissolve diphenyl thiocarbazone (10 mg) in chloroform (1000 ml). Store the solution in glass stoppered, lead free bottle, protected from light and in a refrigerator.

Dilute Standard Lead Solution : Dilute standard lead solution (10.0 ml) (as prepared in heavy metals) with sufficient 1% v/v solution of nitric acid to produce 100 ml. Each ml of this solution contains 1 mg of lead per ml.

Limit Test For Arsenic

In the limit test for arsenic, the amount of arsenic present is expressed as arsenic, As.

Basis of the Test : The pharmacopoeial test of arsenic, which is a toxic component in medicinal substances, is based on the fact that arsenic in the arsenious state can be readily reduced to arsine (AsH_3) gas which on passing over mercuric chloride paper develops a yellow to brown stain, the intensity and length of which are proportional to the amount of arsenic. A standard stain, prepared from a definite amount of arsenic, expresses the limit. Reduction of the arsenic to arsine, both in the sample and the standard, is done by the combined action of zinc, acid, stannous chloride and potassium iodide. The arsine is carried over along with hydrogen to the mercuric chloride or bromide paper supported in the test apparatus. The rate of evolution of hydrogen is controlled which is dependent on the quantity and surface area of zinc, concentration of hydrochloric acid, salt in the reaction mixture, temperature and dimension of the apparatus. Rapid evolution produces a long and diffuse stain while a short and intense colour is developed by a slow evolution.

Chemically, the arsenic impurity is converted in acidic medium into arsenious acid or arsenic acid depending upon the valency state of arsenic :

$$\underset{\text{Trivalent}}{As^{3+}} \longrightarrow \underset{\text{Arsenious acid}}{As(OH)_3 \text{ or } H_3AsO_3}$$

$$\underset{\text{Pentavalent}}{As^{5+}} \longrightarrow \underset{\text{Arsenic acid}}{O = As\ (H)_3 \text{ or } H_3AsO_4}$$

This solution is reacted with a reducing agent like stannous chloride or sulphurous acid to convert the pentavalent arsenic acid into the trivalent arsenious acid which is converted into gaseous arsenious hydride (arsine gas) with the help of nascent hydrogen produced by the action of zinc with hydrochloric acid.

$$\underset{\text{Arsenic acid}}{H_3AsO_4} \longrightarrow \underset{\text{Arsenious acid}}{H_3AsO_3} \xrightarrow[3H]{Zn + HCl} \underset{\text{Arsine}}{AsH_3} + 3H_2O$$

Arsine gas is carried out through the tube with the help of hydrogen to the mercuric chloride paper. Reaction of arsine with mercuric chloride produces a yellow coloured stain. The intensity of the colour is dependent on the quantity of arsenic.

$$2AsH_3 + HgCl_2 \longrightarrow \underset{\text{Yellow}}{Hg(AsH_2)_2} + 2HCl$$

Apparatus

A wide-mouthed flask or bottle capable of holding about 120 ml is fitted with a rubber bung through which passes a glass tube. The latter, made from ordinary glass tubing, has a total length of 200 mm and an internal diameter of exactly 6.5 mm (external diameter about 8 mm). It is drawn out at one end to a diameter of about 1 mm and a hole not less than 2 mm in diameter is blown in the side of the tube, near the constricted part. When the bung is inserted in the bottle containing 70 ml of liquid, the constricted end of the tube is above the surface of the liquid, and the hole in the side is below the bottom of the bung. The upper end of the tube is cut off in square, and is either slightly rounded or ground smooth.

Two rubber bungs (about 25 mm × 25 mm), each with a hole bored centrally and tube, exactly 6.5 mm in diameter, are fitted with a rubber band or spring clip for holding them tightly together. Alternatively the two bungs may be replaced by any suitable contrivance satisfying the conditions.

During the test, the liberated gases pass through the side hole; the lower hole acts as an exit for water which condenses in the tube.

General Method of Testing

By a variable method of procedure, suitable to the particular needs of each substance, a solution is prepared from the substance being examined which may or may not contain that substance, but contains the whole of the arsenic (if any) originally present in that substance. This solution, referred to as the 'test solution', is used in the actual test.

General Test : The glass tube is lightly packed with cotton wool, previously moistened with lead acetate solution and dried, so that the upper surface of the cotton wool is not less than 25 mm below the top of the tube. The upper end of the tube is then inserted into the narrow end of one of the pair of rubber bungs, either to a depth of about 10 mm when the tube has a rounded off end, of the bung. A piece of mercuric chloride paper is placed flat on the top of the bung and the tube is flushed with the larger end of the bung. A piece of mercuric chloride paper is placed flat on the top of the bung and the other bung placed over it and secured by means of the rubber band or spring clip in such a manner that the borings of the two bungs (or the upper bung and the glass tube) meet to form a true tube, 6.5 m in diameter, interrupted by a diaphragm of mercuric chloride paper.

Instead of this method of attaching the mercuric chloride paper, any other method may be used provided (i) that the whole of the evolved gas passes through the paper; (ii) that the portion of the paper in contact with the gas is a circle, 6.5 m in diameter; and (iii) that the paper is protected from sunlight during the test. The test solution prepared as specified, is placed in the wide-mouthed bottle, 1 g of potassium iodide AsT' and 10 g of zinc AsT are added, and the prepared glass tube is placed quickly in position. The action is allowed to proceed for forty minutes. The yellow stain, which is produced on the mercuric chloride paper if arsenic is present, is compared by daylight with the standard stain produced by operating in a similar manner with the known quantities of dilute arsenic solution AsT. The comparison of the stains is made immediately at the completion of the test. The standard stains used for comparison are freshly prepared; they fade on keeping.

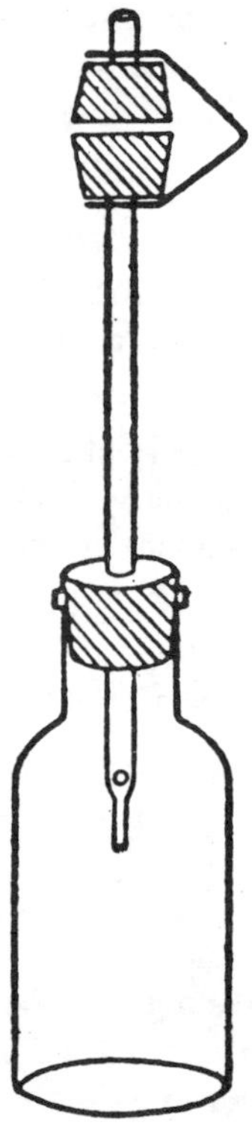

Fig. 7.1 Apparatus for limit test for arsenic

By matching the depth of colour with standard stains, the proportion of arsenic in the substance may be determined. A stain equivalent to the 1 ml standard stain produced by operating on 10 g of a substance indicates that the proportion of arsenic is 1 part per million.

Notes

1. The action may be accelerated by placing the apparatus on a warm surface, care being taken that the mercuric chloride paper remains dry throughout the test.
2. The most suitable temperature for carrying out the test is generally about 40°, but because the rate of evolution of the gas varies somewhat with different batches of zinc

AsT, the temperature may be adjusted to obtain a regular, but not violent, evolution of gas.

3. The tube must be washed with hydrochloric acid AsT, rinsed with water, and dried between successive tests.
4. The stain may be preserved by dipping in hot melted paraffin or placing over phosphorous pentaoxide protected from light. Potassium iodide blackens the stains and makes the comparison easier.
5. Lead acetate papers are used to trap any hydrogen sulphide evolved together with arsine. Hydrogen sulphide reacts with mercuric chloride paper developing a dark stain, thus interfering with the formation of the required mercuric arsenide stain. Metallic zinc may contain traces of sulphide which on reaction with the acid yields hydrogen sulphide.
6. Stannous chloride is required for the complete evolution of arsine. The action between pure zinc and hydrochloric acid is slow and the presence of other metals accelerates the formation of hydrogen. Stannous salts reduce arsenic to arsenious state.

Standard Stains : Solutions are prepared by mixing water (50 ml), stannated hydrochloric acid solution AsT (10 ml) and dilute arsenic solution AsT (varying from 0.2 ml to 1 ml). The resulting solutions, when treated as described in the **General test,** yleld stains, on the mercuric chloride paper referred to as the standard stains.

Reagents and Solutions

Arsenic Solution, dilute AsT :

Strong arsenic solution AsT	1 ml
Water sufficient to produce	100 ml

Dilute arsenic solution AsT must be prepared. One ml of the solution contains 0.01 mg of arsenic. As.

Arsenic Solution, strong, AsT :

Arsenic Trioxide	0.132 g
Hydrochloric acid	50 ml
Water q.s.	100 ml

Brominated hydrochloric acid AsT:

Bromine solution AsT	1 ml
Hydrochloric acid AsT	100 ml

Bromine Solution AsT:

Bromine	30 g
KBr	30 g
Water q.s	100 ml

Mercuric Chloride Paper : Smooth white paper not less than 25 mm in width, soaked in a saturated solution of mercuric chloride, pressed to remove superfluous solution and dried at about 60° in the dark. The grade of the filter paper is such that the weight is between 65 and 120 g per sq mm, the thickness in mm of 400 papers is approximately equal to the weight in g per sq m.

Stannated Hydrochloric Acid AsT

Stannous chloride solution AsT	1 ml
Hydrochloric aeid AsT	100 ml.

Stannous Chloride Solution AsT : Prepared from stannous chloride by adding an equal volume of hydrochloric acid boiling down to the original volume, and filtering through a fine-grain filter paper.

Potassium Iodide AsT : Potassium iodide which complies with the following additional test:

Dissolve the substance (1 g) in hydrochloric acid solution AsT (25 ml) and water (35 ml), add 2 drops of stannous chloride solution AsT and apply the general test, no visible stain is produced.

Citric Acid AsT : Citric acid which complies with the following additional test : Dissolve the substance (10 g) in water (50 ml), add stannated hydrochloric acid solution AsT (10 ml) and apply the general test, no visible stain is produced.

Preparation of the Test Solution

In the various methods of preparing the test solution, the quantities are so arranged, unless otherwise stated, that when the stain produced from the solution to be examined is not deeper than the 1 ml standard stain, the proportion of arsenic present does not exceed the permitted limit.

Modification of the General Testing Method

Some substances require special treatment for performing limit test for arsenic. All the arsenic present in the sample should be present in the final solution in a readily reducible form and the interfering substances should be removed from test sample.

Carbonates, Hydroxides and Oxides

Treatment of carbonates with hydrochloric acid produces carbon dioxide and some hydrochloric acid gas with effervescence and the reaction is exothermic. Oxides and hydroxides on treatment with hydrochloric acid form hydrogen gas with effervescence and evolution of heat. Arsenious chloride ($AsCl_3$) is evolved with hydrochloric acid. If a sample of these substances is treated with hydrochloric acid as such, a part of arsenic may be lost as $AsCl_3$. Therefore, carbonates, oxides and hydroxides are first treated with excess of brominated hydrochloric acid. The bromine oxidizes arsenious to arsenic to the pentavalent form which is not volatile with hydrochloric acid. To perform the test, the arsenic should again be reduced to arsenious state by removing excess of bromine with a few drops of stannous chloride solution.

Sodium Carbonate, Anhydrous, AsT : Anhydrous sodium carbonate which complies with the following additional test : Anhydrous sodium carbonate AsT (5 g) is dissolved in water (50 ml), brominated hydrochloric acid solution AsT (20 ml) is added; the excess of bromine is removed with a few drops of **Stannous chloride solution AsT,** and the General test applied; no visible stain is produced.

Organic Compounds

Most of the organic compounds are insoluble in acid and in water. When gas is evolved in the liquid containing such compounds, undesirable frothing occurs. Therefore, any interfering organic compound should be removed by igniting with anhydrous sodium carbonate before performing the test. Some organic compounds are destroyed by wet oxidation with nitric and sulphuric acids.

Ammonium Oxalate AsT : Ammonium oxalate which complies with the following additional test : Ammonium oxalate (5 g) is heated with water (15 ml), nitric acid solution AsT (5 ml), and sulphuric acid solution AsT (10 ml) in a narrow-necked, round-bottomed flask until frothing ceases, cooled and the General test is applied; no visible stain is produced.

Nitric Acid and Nitrates

Nitric acid and nitrates prevent the reduction of arsenic which are removed by heating the substance with concentrated sulphuric acid and evaporating nitric acid off. Arsenic is left in the sulphuric acid. The remaining traces of nitric acid are removed by diluting residual sulphuric acid with water and re-evaporating the mixture. Now the nitrosylsulphuric acid formed during first evaporation is decomposed and the sulphuric acid becomes free from nitric acid. Solution of ferric chloride also contains some nitric acid which is also removed by the similar treatment.

Nitric Acid AsT : Nitric acid which complies with the following additional test : Nitric acid solution AsT (20 ml) heated in a porcelain dish with sulphuric acid AsT (2 ml) until white fumes are given off. It is cooled, water (2 ml) is added and again heated until white fumes are given off. It is cooled, water (50 ml) and stannated hydrochloric acid AsT (10 ml) are added and the General test is applied; no visible stain is produced.

Boric Acid and Borax

Boric acid is slightly soluble in hydrochloric acid, but it is dissolved along with citric acid. Borax is converted into boric acid on treatment with hydrochloric acid. Therefore, citric acid is added to dissolve boric acid and borax before addition of stannated hydrochloric acid.

Ammonia Solution

Solutions are heated on a water bath to remove the free ammonia. Arsenic is left as ammonium arsenate and arsenite in the solution which are acidified with brominated hydrochloric acid and stannous chloride is added.

Liquid Glucose and Potassium Acid Tartrate

Liquid glucose often contains traces of sulphur dioxide as preservative while sulphite are present in potassium acid tartrate. These substances are treated with brominated hydrochloric acid to oxidize the sulphurous acid. Excess of bromine is removed by adding few drops of stannous chloride solution.

Hypophosphorus Acid

Reduction of hypophosphorus acid yields phosphine which interacts with mercuric halide papers. Hence, it is oxidized to phosphoric acid by treating with potassium chlorate and hydrochloric acid. Excess of chloride formed by the reaction of chlorate and hydrochloric acid is removed by boiling and then by treating with stannous chloride.

Oxidizing Agents

The oxidizing agents such as potassium chlorate should be completely reduced, otherwise, whole of the hydrogen will be utilized to reduce the substance and arsine would not be evolved.

Potassium Chlorate AsT : Potassium chlorate which complies with the following additional test : The substance (5 g) is mixed in the cold with water (20 ml) and hydrochloric acid solution AsT (22 ml) is added; when the first reaction has subsided, heat gently to expel chlorine, the last traces are removed with a few drops of stannous chloride solution AsT; water (20 ml) added, and the General test is applied; no visible stain is produced.

Compounds of Copper, Bismuth, Antimony and Iron

Copper deposits on zinc forming a zinc-copper mixture which interfere in the steady evolution of hydrogen and all the arsenic will not convert into arsine. Bismuth deposits on zinc forming a solid sponge-like mass preventing evolution of hydrogen. Antimony compounds form antimony hydride with nascent hydrogen which produces a dark stain on mercuric chloride paper interfering with the stain developed due to arsine. Iron also reduces the rate of evolution of hydrogen and arsenic is not reduced completely to arsine.

Copper, bismuth and iron salts are treated with dilute hydrochloric acid (20%) and distilled. Whole of the arsenic present in the substance distils in the first 75% distillate. Sufficient stannous chloride is added to reduce ferric salts to ferrous state.

A double distillation is required to perform the test of antimony compounds since antimony is slightly volatile in hydrochloric acid.

Sulphur

Sulphur is present as arsenic sulphide which is soluble in ammonium sulphide and ammonia. Therefore, sulphur is digested with ammonia to form ammonium polysulphides in which arsenic sulphide is soluble. The mixture is filtered to separate undissolved sulphur and the filtrate dried. The residue containing arsenic and some sulphur is treated with anhydrous sodium carbonate and water. Sodium polysulphide is formed in which arsenic sulphide is soluble. The solution is boiled and bromine added to oxidize arsenic to arsenate and sulphide to sulphate. The solution is acidified, boiled and treated with stannous chloride to perform the General tests.

8

Detection of Nitrogen, Sulphur and Halogen Elements in Organic Compounds

Organic compounds are non-ionic in nature. Therefore, they are fused with sodium metal for detection of these elements to convert them into inorganic compounds (ionized form). Based on this fact, Lassaigne's test was developed by J.L. Lassaigne.

Lassiagne's Test

Insert a small piece of freshly cut, clean and dry sodium into an ignition tube followed by addition of organic compound. Heat the ignition tube in a bunsen flame gently till sodium melts and then strongly till it becomes red hot. The red hot ignition tube is immediately plunged into a porcelain dish containing distilled water (50 ml). Two or three ignition tubes are added into water in the same way. Crush the tube by gentle tapping, boil the solution for 30 minutes and then filtered. The filtrate is known as sodium extract. In this way, nitrogen is converted into inorganic cyanide while the halogens and sulphur formed halides and sulphide, respectively.

$$Na + C + N \longrightarrow NaCN$$

$$2Na + X_2 \longrightarrow 2NaX \quad (X = Cl^-, Br^-, I^-)$$

$$2Na + S \longrightarrow Na_2S$$

The above sodium extract is alkaline in nature due to formation of sodium hydroxide.

$$Na + 2H_2O \longrightarrow 2NaOH + H_2 \uparrow$$

Test for Nitrogen

Take the above sodium extract (2 or 3 ml) into a test tube containing powdered ferrous sulphate crystals about 0.2 g. Boil the solution gently and then add just sufficient dilute sulphuric acid to dissolve the iron hydroxides and make the solution acidic. Formation of Prussian blue precipitate or colour indicates the presence of nitrogen.

$$\underset{\text{Ferrous sulphate}}{FeSO_4} + NaOH \longrightarrow Fe(OH)_2 \downarrow + Na_2SO_4$$

$$Fe(OH)_2 + 6NaCN \longrightarrow \underset{\substack{\text{Sodium ferrocyanide} \\ \text{(Prussian blue)}}}{Na_4[Fe(CN)_6]} + 2NaOH.$$

Test for Sulphur

(i) Sodium Nitroprusside Test : Add few drops of freshly prepared dilute solution of sodium nitroprusside, $Na_2[Fe(CN)_5 NO]2H_2O$, to the sodium extract (2 ml). Formation of purple colour confirms the presence of sulphur.

$$\underset{\text{(Sodium extract)}}{Na_2S} + Na_2[Fe(CN)_5 NO] \longrightarrow \underset{\text{Purple coluor}}{Na_4[Fe(CN)_5 NOS]}$$

(ii) Lead Acetate Test : Acidity the sodium extract (2 ml) with dilute acetic acid and then add lead acetate solution. Formation of black precipitate of lead sulphide confirms the presence of sulphur.

$$Na_2S + \underset{\text{Lead acetate}}{Pb(CH_3COO)_2O} \longrightarrow \underset{\text{Lead sulphide (black)}}{PbS} + 2CH_3COONa.$$

Test for Nitrogen and Sulphur

If the organic compound contains nitrogen and sulphur together, then sodium thiocyanate is formed during fusion with sodium. Sodium thiocyanate gives a blood red colour with ferric chloride solution.

$$Na + S + N + C \xrightarrow{\text{Fusion}} \underset{\text{Sodium sulphocyanide}}{NaCNS}$$

$$3NaCNS + FeCl_3 \longrightarrow Fe(CNS)_3 + 3NaCl$$

Ferric sulphocyanide (Blood red colour)

Test for Chloride, Bromide and Iodide

Take sodium extract (5 ml) and add dilute HNO_3 solution to it. Boil the solution to expel H_2S or HCN, if present, and then add few drops of silver nitrate solution.

(i) Formation of white precipitate, soluble in NH_4OH, indicates the presence of chloride in the organic compound.

(ii) Pale yellow precipitate, soluble in excess of NH_4OH, shows the presence of bromide.

(iii) Yellow precipitate, insoluble in NH_4OH, confirms the presence of iodide.

$$NaX + \underset{\text{Silver nitrate}}{AgNO_3} \xrightarrow{\text{dil } HNO_3} AgX\downarrow + NaNO_3$$

Silver halide ($X = Cl^-, Br, I$)

$$\underset{\text{White ppt}}{AgCl} + \underset{\text{Ammonia}}{2NH_4OH} \longrightarrow [Ag(NH_3)_2]^+ Cl^- + 2H_2O$$

Silver aminochloride (soluble)

$$\underset{\text{Pale yellow ppt}}{AgBr} + 2NH_4OH \longrightarrow [Ag(NH_3)_2]^+Br^- + 2H_2O$$

Slightly soluble

$$\underset{\text{Yellow ppt}}{AgI} + NH_4OH \longrightarrow \text{No reaction.}$$

9

Determination of Melting and Boiling Points

Melting point of solid or boiling point of any liquid are determined in order:

(i) to check purity of the substances. Pure substances have sharp and definite melting point/boiling point. The impure substance melts slowly. Similarly, boiling point of the impure liquid is high.

(ii) to identify the organic compounds. If the m.p. or b.p. of the given organic compound is determined with an accuracy of $\pm 2^{\circ}$, then possible compound can easily be guessed.

Method of Determination of Melting Point

A thin capillary of about 5 cm in length with uniform bore is sealed at one end by bringing it near the flame. The pure, dry and fine powdered compound (nearly 2 mg) under indentification is filled through open end of the capillary tube by gentle tapping the closed end.

Fix the assembly as shown in the Fig. (9.1) which is consisted of a long necked flask (heating bath) containing concentrated sulphuric acid, glycerol or liquid paraffin (It is safer to use liquid paraffin). Moist the filled capillary with the liquid of flask and place it along side of thermometer with it sealed end near the bulb of thermameter. The capillary tube will cling to the thermometer by capillary attraction. The flask is then heated gently by holding the burner in hand and rotating the flame round the bottom of flask so that the temperature of liquid rises uniformly. Observe the temperature and organic compound closely and record the temperature when substance begins to melt and become transparent. Repeat the experiment to determine the melting point as accurately as possible.

Method of Determination of Boiling Point

The liquid (0.5 ml) of which boiling point is to be determined is taken in the ignition tube and tied with the thermometer by mean of rubber or thread. The thermameter along with ignition tube is fixed in the heating bath as shown is the Fig. (9.2). A sealed capillary tube, as in determination in melting point, is put into ignition tube containing liquid. Keep the fused end dipped in the liquid. Heat the bath gently and uniformly. The air bubbles from the end of the capillary tube start escaping at a slow rate but when the boiling point of the liquid is attained, a continuous escape of air bubbles will be observed. This temperature is recorded, and heating discontinued. The temperature is again recorded when the last air bubble appears. This temperature is the point at which the vapour pressure of the liquid is equal to atmospheric pressure. The mean of these two readings is the accurate boiling point of the liquid. This operation may be repeated for accuracy.

If the boiling point obtained is the same for second time also, the liquid is considered to be pure and easy to identify.

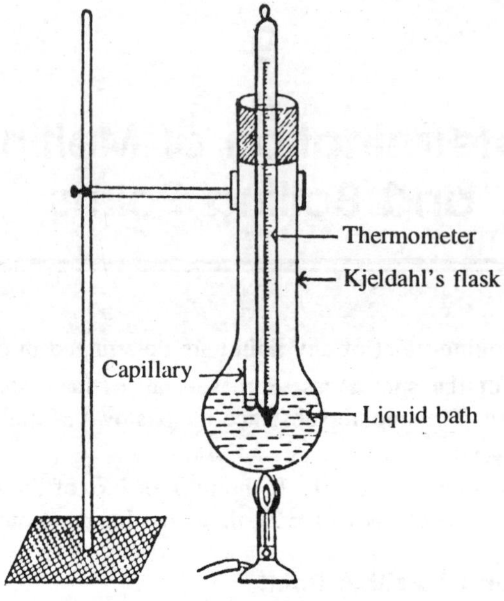

Fig. 9.1 Determination of Melting Point

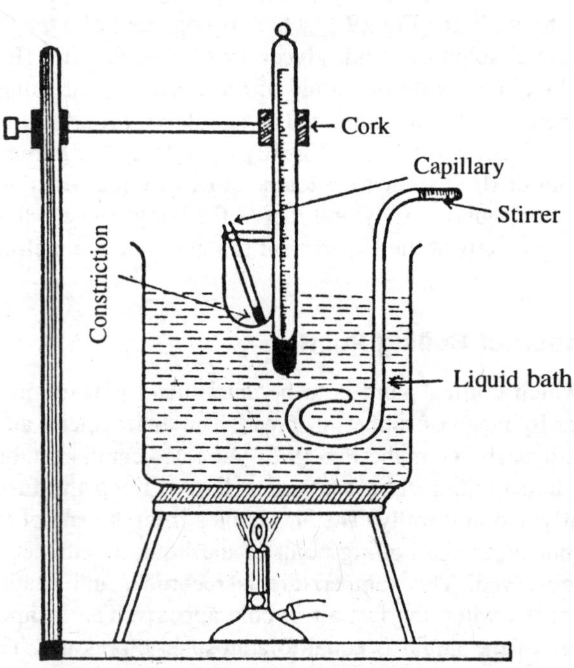

Fig. 9.2 Determination of Boiling Point

10

Qualitative Organic Analysis

It includes the systematic identification of an organic compound. An unknown organic compound can be identified by the following steps:

1. Physical examination of the compound.
2. Tests for unsaturation
3. Solubility tests
4. Detection of elements
5. Detection of functional groups.
6. Determination of melting point or boiling point of the compound.
7. Confirmatory tests of the inferred organic compound
8. Preparation of derivatives and determination of their melting points.

1. Physical Examination of the Compound

The following physical characters are helpful in identifying the compounds:

(i) Colour : Organic compounds are coloured due to the presence of a chromophoric group. Sometimes compound can be guessed by observing the colour as show below.

Pale yellow — Nitro compounds, iodoform.

Orange — o-Nitroaniline, alizarin, phenanthroquinone, azo compounds.

Red — 1, 2–Napthoquinone.

(ii) Odour : The presence of characteristic odours is an indicative of a particular class, of organic compounds.

Pleasant — Esters, ether, lower aliphatic alcohols, chloroform.

Bitter almonds — Nitrobenzene, benzaldehyde.

Phenolic — Phenols, naphthols, some derivatives of salicylic acid.

Pungent — Acetic acid, acetyl chloride, acetic anhydride, benzoyl chloride, benzyl chloride, formic acid and pyridine

Moth balls : Naphthalene.

Fishy - Amines.

Rotten eggs : Sulphur containing compounds.

(iii) Ignition : A small amount of compound is kept on spatula and burnt in a flame. The original compound can be predicted on the basis of behaviour. Smoky flame indicates aromatic compounds while aliphatic compounds burn with non-smoky flame. Polyhalogenated compounds generally do not ignite. Compounds such as carbohydrates, tartaric acid and its salts are charred on ignition. Iodoform burns with violet vapours.

2. Tests for unsaturation

To find out the unsaturation, the following tests are performed:

(i) Bromine Test ; To a solution of compound, bromine solution is added dropwise with shaking. Disappearance of reddish brown colour of bromine solution indicates unsaturation.

(ii) Baeyer Test : To a solution of organic compound in water or ethanol, Beayer's reagent (1% $KMnO_4$ solution) is added dropwise with continuous shaking. The disappearance of purple colour also indicates the presence of unsaturated compound.

3. Solubility Tests

Solubility behaviour of the organic compound can provide valuable information regarding the presence or absence of certain classes of organic compounds. Therefore, it should be checked.

Generally the solubility test is performed in the following sequence:

(i) Dissolve the organic compound (100 mg) in water (3-5 ml) with shaking. If the compound dissolves, then repeat the test with ether as solvent.

(ii) When the compound is insoluble in water, observe its solubility in 5% NaOH solution. If it is soluble in sodium hydroxide, test its solubility in 5% $NaHCO_3$ solution.

(iii) The compound, insoluble in sodium hydroxide solution, is further checked for its solubility in 5% HCl.

(iv) An organic compound, which remained insoluble in water, NaOH and HCl solution, contains no nitrogen again is tested for its solubility in concentrated H_2SO_4

The Table 10.1 gives the solubility classes of various organic compound on which basis conclusion regarding the presence or absence of some classes can be drawn.

4. Detection of Elements

Organic compounds are consisted of two or more elements. Generally they contain carbon and hydrogen but the presence of nitrogen, sulphur and halogen is determined in certain compound (see Chapter 8).

5. Detection of Functional Groups

Functional group analysis is performed in the following order:

(A) Compounds Containing C and H With or Without Oxygen.

(a) Carboxylic Group , —COOH

(i) **Litmus Paper Test :** Solution of organic compounds gives red colour with blue litmus paper.

(ii) **Sodium Bicarbonate Test :** To a saturated solution of sodium bicarbonate in a test tube, a small quantity of the compound is added. Evolution of CO_2 with brisk effervescences indicates the presence of carboxylic group.

$$\underset{\text{Carboxylic acid.}}{R\text{—}COOH} + NaHCO_3 \longrightarrow \underset{\text{Sodium salt}}{R\text{-}COO^-Na^+} + H_2O + CO_2 \uparrow$$

(iii) **Ester Formation** : Heat gently ethanol (1 ml) with the compound (0.5 g or 1 ml) and a few drops of concentrated sulphuric acid for about one minute in a testtube. A fruity odour of ester indicates the presence of carboxylic group.

$$\underset{\text{Carboxylic acid.}}{R\text{—}COOH} + \underset{\text{Ethanol}}{C_2H_5OH} \xrightleftharpoons[\text{heat}]{\text{Conc. } H_2SO_4} \underset{\text{Ester}}{R\text{—}COOC_2H_5} + H_2O$$

Table 10.1. Classification of Organic Compounds According to Solubility.

Soluble in Both Ether and Water	Soluble in Water but Insoluble in Ether	Soluble in 5% sodium Hydroxide Solution	Soluble in 5% Hydrochloric Acid	Not Containing N or S; soluble only in Concentrated Sulphuric Acid	Not Containing N or S. Insoluble in Concentrated Sulphuric Acid	Containing N or S. Compounds not covered in previous categories
The lower members of the homologous series of : 1. Alcohols 2. Aldehydes 3. Ketones 4. Acids 5. Esters 6. Phenols 7. Anhydrides 8. Amines 9. Nitriles 10. Polyhydroxy Phenols	1. Polybasic acids and hydroxy acids. 2. Glycols, polyhydric alcohols polyhydroxy aldehydes and ketones (sugars) 3. Some amides, amino acids, di- and polyamino compounds 4. Sulphonic acids 5. Sulphonic acids salts.	1. Acids 2. Phenols 3. Imides 4. Some primary and secondary nitro com pounds; oximes 5. Mercaptans and thiophenols 6. Sulphonic acids, sul phamic acids, and sul phonamides 7. Some diketones and β-keto esters	1. Primary amines 2. Secondary aliphatic and aryl alkyl amines 3. Aliphatic and some aryl-alkyl tertiary amines 4. Hydrazines.	1. Unsaturated hydrocarbons 2. Some polyalky lated aromatic hydrocarbons 3. Alcohols 4. Aldehydes 5. Ketones 6. Esters 7. Anhydrides 8. Ethers and acetals 9. Lactones 10. Acylhalides	1. Saturated aliphatic hydrocarbons 2. Cyclic paraffin hydrocarbons 3. Aromatic hydrocarbons 4. Halogen derivatives of 1, 2 and 3 5. Diaryl ethers	1. Nitro com pounds 2. Amides and derivatives of aldehydes and ketones 3. Nitriles 4. Negatively substituted amines 5. Nitroso, azo, hydrazo, and other inter mediate reduction products of nitro compounds 6. Sulphones, sulphonamides of secondary amines, sul phides, sul phates and other sulphur compounds.

(b) Alcoholic group, – OH

(i) To a solution of organic compound, add few drops of ceric ammonium nitrate reagent. Appearance of red colour confirms the presence of alcoholic group.

$$\underset{\text{Alcohol}}{2ROH} + \underset{\text{Ceric ammonium nitrate}}{(NH_4)_2\,Ce(NO_3)_6} \longrightarrow \underset{\text{Red complex}}{(ROH)_2\,Ce\,(NO_3)_4} + 2NH_4\,NO_3.$$

(ii) **Sodium Test (for Liquid only) :** To organic compound (2 ml), add a small piece of sodium metal. Vigorous effervescences due to liberation of hydrogen gas indicate the presence of alcoholic hydroxy group.

$$2ROH + 2Na \longrightarrow 2\,RONa + H_2\uparrow$$

(iii) **Ester Test :** To a solution of organic compound, add few drops of acetic acid and a drop of concentrated H_2SO_4 and heat gently. Fruity odour of ester indicates the presence of alcoholic group.

$$\underset{\text{Alcohol}}{ROH} + \underset{\text{Acetic acid}}{CH_3COOH} \underset{\text{heat}}{\overset{H_2SO_4}{\rightleftharpoons}} \underset{\text{Ester}}{CH_3COOR} + H_2O$$

(c) Phenolic Group (– OH directly attached to an aromatic nucleus)

(i) **Litmus Paper Test :** The solution of phenolic compounds turns blue litmus to red.

(ii) **Ferric Chloride Test :** To a solution of phenol (1 ml), add few drops of 5% ferric chloride solution. Violet, green, pink or red colour is appeared due to formation of the phenol complex ion.

$$6\,C_6H_5OH + FeCl_3 \longrightarrow \underset{\text{Complexion (coloured)}}{[Fe\,(OC_6H_5)_6\,]^{3-}} + HCl + 3H^+$$

(iii) **Liebermann's Nitroso Reaction :** Dissolve an organic compound (0.1 g) in concentrated sulphuric acid (1 ml) in a dry test tube and add few crystals of sodium nitrite. A blue-green or blue-violet colour is appeared which changes to red on dilution with water. This colour changes to green, blue or violet on addition of sodium hydroxide solution. (This test is only performed with the organic compound having free phenolic group at para position)

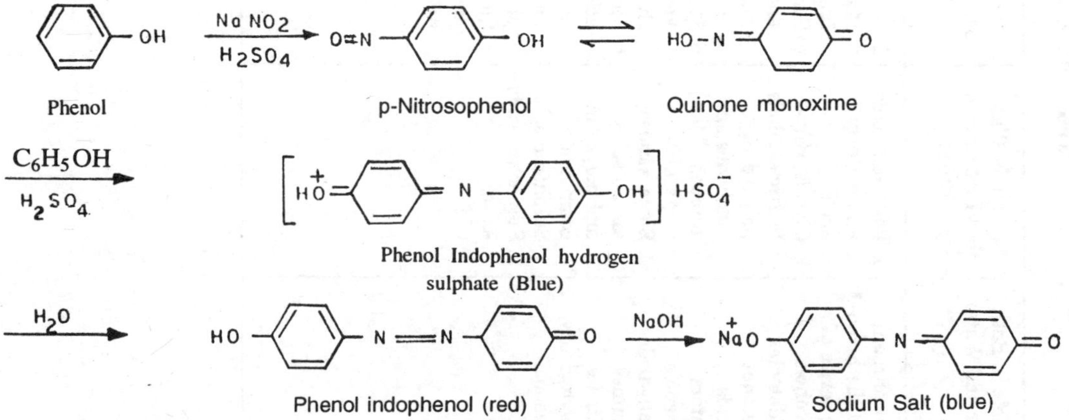

(iv) **Phthalein Test :** Heat the organic compound (0.2 g) and phthalic anhydride with concentrated sulphuric acid (2 drops) for one minute. Cool it and pour the contents into a beaker containing sodium hydroxide. The following characteristic colours are obtained:

Phenol	—	Red
Catechol, hydroquinone	—	Blue
Naphthols	—	Light green
p-Cresol	—	Colourless

(v) **Azo Dye Test :** Cool down a mixture of few drops of aniline, little sodium nitrite and dilute hydrochloric acid (1 ml) in freezing bath below 4°C. Add an alkaline solution of organic compound to it. Formation of orange dye indicates the presence of phenol.

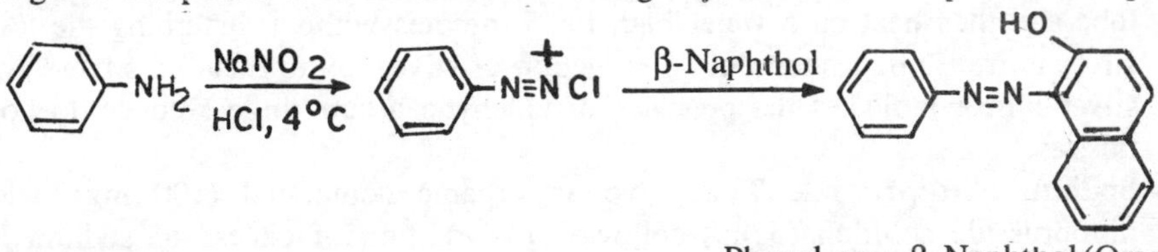

Phenyl azo–β-Naphthol (Orange dye)

(d) Carbonyl Group , $>C=O$

The carbonyl group is present in aldehyde, $-\overset{H}{C}=O$ and ketonic group, $>C=O$. Both these group are detected by the following test.

(i) **2, 4–Dinitrophenylhydrazine Test :** To 2, 4 - dinitrophenylhydrazine solution (2 ml), add organic compound with vigorous shaking. Appearance of orange or red precipitate indicates the presence of carbonyl group.

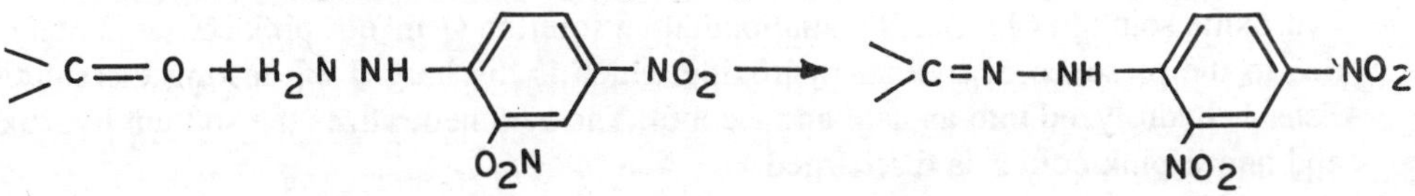

2, 4-Dinitrophenyl hydrazine Phenylazo-β - Naphthol (orange dye)

(ii) **Sodium Bisulphite Test :** To a sodium bisulphite solution (3 ml), add organic compound (100 mg). Formation of white precipitate shows the presence of carbonyl group.

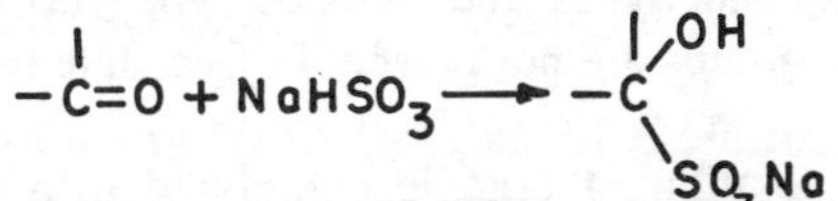

Bisulphite compound (white precipitate)

Differentiation Between Aldehyde and Ketonic Groups

(i) **Schiff's Reaction :** To Schiff's reagent (2 ml), add few drops of the organic compound. A deep violet-red or red colour indicates the presence of aldehyde group. The test is negative in ketonic and some aromatic aldehydes (eg. vanillin).

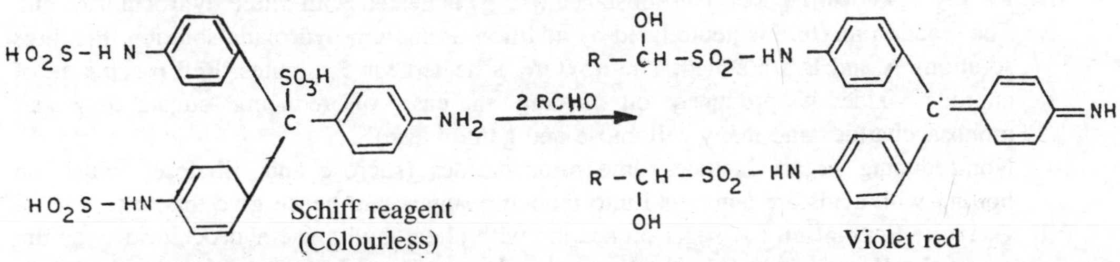

Schiff reagent (Colourless) Violet red

(ii) **Fehling's Solution Test :** Only aldehydes reduce Fehling's solution to red cuprous oxide. Mix 1 ml of each Fehling's solutions A and B in a test tube and add a small amount of organic compound to it. Boil the solution for 5 minutes on a water bath. Formation of reddish brown precipitate of cuprous oxide (Cu_2O) indicates the persence of aldehyde group.

$$R-\overset{\displaystyle H}{\overset{|}{C}}=O + 2CuO \longrightarrow RCOOH + \underset{\text{Cuprous oxide (Red ppt.)}}{Cu_2O}$$

(iii) **Tollen's Test :** Add 10% sodium hydroxide solution (1 ml) to a freshly prepared 10% silver nitrate solution (1 ml) with shaking. To the mixture, add NH_4OH solution till the precipitated substance just dissolves. Add little organic compound along the sides of tube and then heat on a water bath for 5 minutes without disturbing the test tube. A silver mirror is deposited due to reduction of silver ion to metallic silver. The shining silver mirror indicates the presence of aldehyde group while ketones do not respond this test.

(iv) **Sodium Nitroprusside Test :** To an organic compound (100 mg), add sodium nitroprusside solution (5 ml) followed by addition of excess of sodium hydroxide solution. Formation of red colour indicates the presence of ketonic group. This test in negative in case of aldehydes and aromatic ketones.

(e) Ester Group $\left(R-\overset{\displaystyle O}{\overset{\|}{C}}-OR^1\right)$

(i) **Fruity Smell :** All the esters have fruity smell.

(ii) **Phenolphthalein Test :** To the organic compound (100 mg), add dilute sodium hydroxide solution (3 ml) and phenolphthalein solution (1 ml). A pink colour is obtained due to the presence of sodium hydroxide which is discharged on heating the solution. Ester is hydrolyzed into an acid and alcohol. The acid neutralizes the sodium hydroxide and hence pink colour is discharged.

$$R_1-COOR_2 + H_2O \xrightarrow{NaOH} R_1-COOH + R_2OH$$

(f) Carbohydrates

Carbohydrates are polyhydroxy aldehydes and ketones. They do not give all the tests of aldehydic or ketonic group as these groups are not present in free state in the carbohydrates. They are detected by following tests.

(i) **Molisch's Test :** To a solution of organic compound in a test tube, add Molisch's reagent (10% alcoholic solution of α-naphthol) with shaking. Pour concentrated sulphuric acid solution (2 ml) along the side of inclined tube carefully so that the acid forms a layer beneath the aqueous solution without mixing. Appearance of deep violet ring at the junction of two liquids indicates the presence of carbohydrate. This colour becomes violet-red on shaking the contents.

(ii) **Felling's Solution Test :** The substance (0.5 g) is heated with dilute hydrochloric acid. The reaction mixture is neutralized by addition of sodium hydroxide solution. Fehlings solutions A and B are added. The mixture is heated for 5 minutes. Red precipitate of cuprous oxide is produced on heating in case of reducing sugars (e.g. all monosaccharides and many cellobiose and gentiobiose).

Non-reducing sugars include some disaccharides (sucrose and trihalose) which on boiling with acids are converted into reducing sugars and hence give this test.

(iii) **Osazone Formation :** A sugar on heating with phenylhydrazine hydrochloride, sodium acetate and acetic acid forms yellow crystals of osazone. Monosaccharides (reducing sugars only) form osazones.

CHO		CH_2OH	$CH = N\text{-}NH\ C_6H_5$
|		|	|
CHOH	or	$C = 0 + 2C_6H_5NHNH_2 \longrightarrow$	$C = N.NHC_6H_5$
|		|	|
$(CHOH)_3$		$(CHOH)_3$	$(CHOH)_3$
|		|	|
CH_2OH		CH_2OH	CH_2OH
Glucose		Fructose	Osazone

Take the compound (0.2 g) with phenylhydrazine hydrochloride (0.5 g), sodium acetate (0.5 g) and water (5 ml). Boil them on a water bath with occasional shaking till precipitate appears (Note the time of osazone formation). It is cooled and filtered.

(iv) **Resorcinol Test for Ketones (Selivanoff's Test) :** A crystal of resorcinol is added to the solution and heated with an equal volume of concentrated hydrochloric acid. Pink colour is formed in case of ketoses (e.g. fructose).

Differentiation Between Monosaccharides and Disaccharides

Heat the Barfoed's reagent with aqueous solution of organic compound on a water bath. If red colour due to formation of cuprous oxide is developed readily, a monosaccharide (glucose, fructose) is present. Disaccharides, e.g. sucrose may develop the red colour on prolonged heating (about 10 minutes) due to partial hydrolysis into monosaccharides.

(g) Hydrocarbons

Hydrocarbons may be saturated and unsaturated. Unsaturated hydrocarbon may be aliphatic or aromatic in nature. They are insoluble in water but soluble in many organic solvents. Due to lack of reactivity, their identification is based on result of preliminary tests (test of unsaturation, detection of elements), determination of melting point/boiling point, specific test for particular hydrocarbons and preparation of their derivatives.

(h) Ethers

After performing the above steps and if the compound do not contain extra element, there may be possibility of ethers which are tested as follows:

(i) **Feigl's Test :** Heat the substance (2 ml) after covering the mouth of test tube with a filter paper moistened with a mixture of cupric acetate and benzidine hydrocloride; a deep blue colour appears on the filter paper.

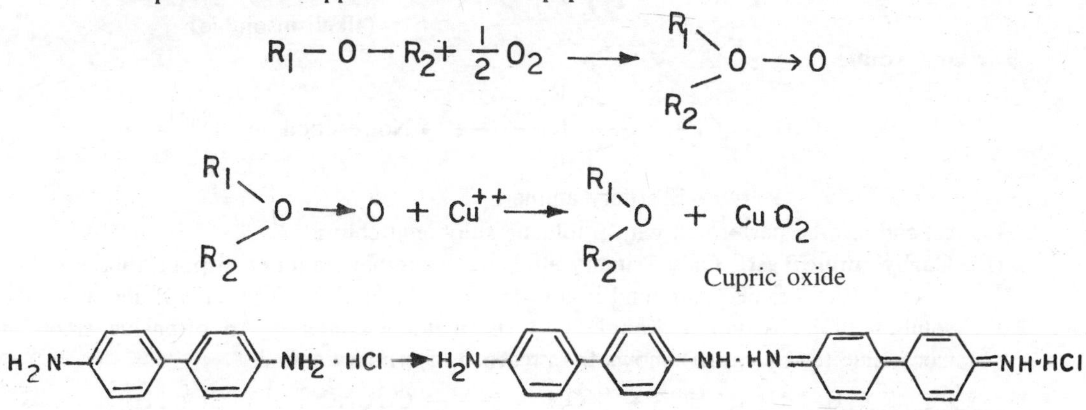

(Benzidine blue)

(ii) Dissolve 2 or 3 drops of the substance in benzene (5 ml). Add very dilute solution of iodine in benzene (5 ml) and shake, a brown tint appears.

(B) Compounds Containing C, H, N with or without Oxygen Atom.

(a) Amino Group.

It may be primary ($-NH_2$), secondary ($-\overset{|}{N}H$) and tertiary ($-N<$) group.

(i) **Hinsberg Test :** This test is performed to differentiate the primary, secondary and tertiary amines.

To an organic compound (0.1 g), add benzene sulphonyl chloride (0.2 g) and 10% sodium hydroxide solution (5 ml) with vigorous shaking. Observe the formation of precipitate of benzene sulphonyl derivative. If no reaction to occur, heat the contents on a water bath for 2-3 minutes and then cool in ice.

On cooling if no solid separates out, the organic compound may betertiary amine. If a precipitate appears in alkaline medium, add water (5 ml) with shaking. If the precipitate does not dissolve, it indicates the presence of secondary amines.

In case of clear solution, acidify with dilute hydrochloric acid. Appearance of a precipitate indicates the persence of primary amine.

Primary Amine:

$$C_6H_5SO_2Cl + H_2NR \xrightarrow{NaOH} C_6H_5SO_2N(Na)R$$

Benzene sulphonyl Chloride; Primary amine; Benzene sulphonyl derivative (Water soluble)

$$\downarrow HCl$$

$$C_6H_5SO_2NHR$$

Benzene sulphonyl derivative (Water insoluble)

Secondary Amine:

$$C_6H_5SO_2Cl + HN\begin{matrix} R_1 \\ R_2 \end{matrix} \xrightarrow{NaOH} C_6H_5SO_2N\begin{matrix} R_1 \\ R_2 \end{matrix}$$

Secondary amine; Benzene sulphonyl derivative (alkali insoluble)

Tertiary Amine

$$C_6H_5SO_2Cl + N\begin{matrix} R_1 \\ R_2 \\ R_3 \end{matrix} \longrightarrow \text{No reaction}$$

Tertiary amine

This test can also be performed with p-toluene sulphonyl chloride.

(ii) **Carbylamine Test :** Only Primary aliphatic or aromatic amines respond this test. Take a little organic compound in a test tube and add chloroform (1 ml) and alcoholic solution of potassium hydroxide (2 ml). Heat the contents. An offensive smell of isocyanide (carbylamine) shows the presence of primary amine.

$$C_6H_5NH_2 + CHCl_3 + 3KOH \longrightarrow C_6H_5NC \uparrow + 3KCl + 3H_2O.$$

Aniline; Phenyl isocyanide (Carbylamine)

(iii) **Azo Dye Test :** If the carbylamine test is positive, then azo dye test is performed to determine whether the amine is primary aliphatic or aromatic one.

Dissolve organic compound (0.5 g) in dilute hydrochloric acid (5 ml). Cool down the solution in ice bath below 4°C. Add slowly sodium nitrite (0.5 g) and dissolved in water (5 ml) with shaking. Now add a few drops of an alkaline solution of β - naphthol. Formation of yellow, orange or red dye confirms a primary aromatic amine.

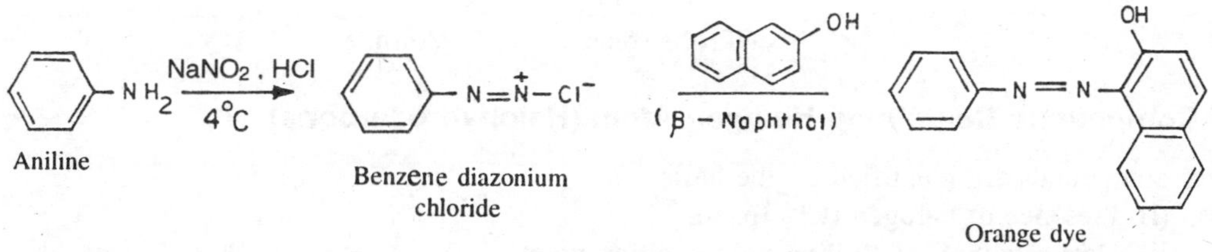

(b) Primary Amide Group

(i) Heat organic compound (0.2 g) with 10% sodium hydroxide solution (2 ml) in a test tube. Evolution of ammonia indicates the presence of an amide group. Formation of ammonia is detected by dense white fumes with glass rod dipped in concentrated hydrochloric acid.

(c) Anilide Group (-NHCOR)

(i) **Tafel's Test :** Add concentrated sulphuric acid (3 ml) and potassium dichromate (0.3 g) to a little organic compound in a test tube. Red or violet colour changing to green shows the presence of anilide which do not contain substituent in the benzene nucleus.

(ii) **2, 4-Dinitrochlorobenzene Test :** Organic compound having anilide group gives intense colour on a paper soaked with 2, 4-dinitrochlorobenzene.

(iii) **Azo Dye Test :** It also undergoes diazotization and coupling in the same way as primary amines to form azo dye.

(d) Nitro Group $\left(-\text{N}\begin{matrix} \nearrow\!\!\!\!/\,\text{O} \\ \searrow \text{O} \end{matrix} \right)$

(i) **Tollen's reagent test :** To the organic compound (0.5 g) in ethanol (10 ml) in a test tube, add ammonium chloride (0.5 g) and zinc dust (0.5 g) with shaking. Heat the contents on a water bath for 5 minutes. Cool the mixture, filter and add ammonical solution of silver nitrate (Tollen's reagent) (1 ml). Formation of silver mirror indicates the presence of nitro group.

$$\underset{\text{Nitrobenzene}}{C_6H_5NO_2} \xrightarrow[NH_4Cl]{\text{Zinc}} \underset{\text{Phenyl hydroxylamine}}{C_6H_5NHOH} + H_2O$$

$$C_6H_5OH + 2\,[Ag(NH_3)_2]OH \longrightarrow C_6H_5NO + \underset{\text{(Silver mirror)}}{2Ag^+} + 4NH_3 + 2H_2O$$

(ii) **Ferrous Hydroxide Test :** Add an organic compound (0.1 g) to a solution of 5% ferrous ammonium sulphate in a test tube. Then add 3 drops of 6N sulphuric acid followed by 2N potassium hydroxide solution (2 ml) in methanol. Formation of red brown precipitate indicates the presence of nitro group.

$$R - NO_2 + \underset{\text{Blue green}}{6\ Fe\ (OH)_2} \longrightarrow + \underset{\text{Brown.}}{6Fe\ (OH)_3}$$

(iii) **Azo Dye Test :** To the organic compound (1 ml), add zinc and concentrated HCl and then boil the contents for 5 minutes in a boiling tube. Nitro group is converted into amino group and then usual azo dye test can be performed as in the case of primary amino group.

$$C_6H_5NO_2 \xrightarrow[HCl]{Zn} C_6H_5NH_2$$

Nitrobenzene Aniline

(C) Compounds Containing Halogen Atom (Halohydrocarbons)

These compounds are identified on the basis of:

(i) Presence of halogen (Cl^-, Br^-, or I^-)
(ii) Determination of Boiling point/melting point.
(iii) Preparation of suitable derivatives
(iv) Determination of Boiling point/melting point of derivative.

The reactivity of halogen derivatives is tested by silver nitrate. The organic compound is heated with an alcoholic solution of silvers nitrate. If white or yellow precipitate is obtained, it indicates the presence of halogen in the side chain. A halogen atom directly attached to an aromatic nucleus like chlorobenzene does not react with silver nitrate solution.

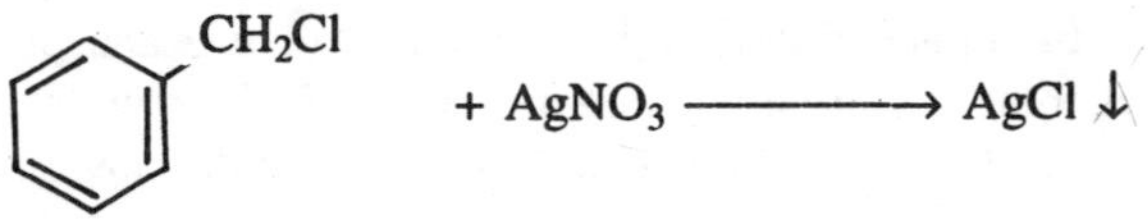

Benzyl chloride — White precipitate

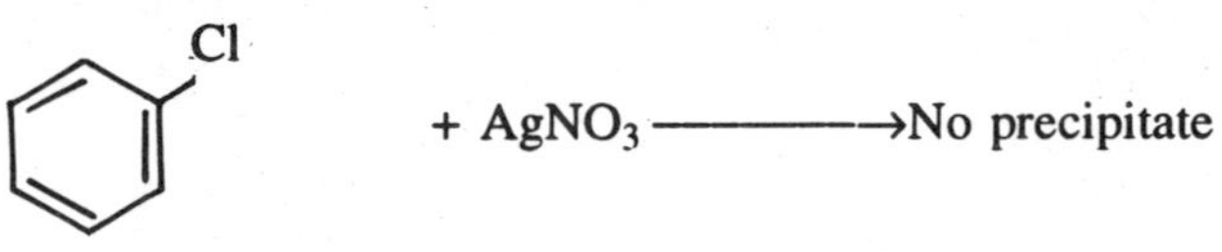

Chlorobenzene

(D) Compounds Containing C, H and Sulphur with Oxygen or without Oxygen.

(a) Sulphonic Acids (—SO_3 H)

Test of this group is performed if sulphur is present and compound gives brisk effervescence with sodium bicarbonate

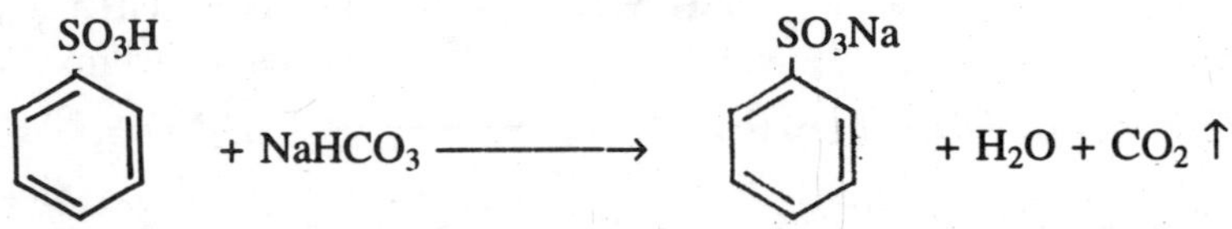

(i) **Potassium Hydroxide Fusion Test :** Heat organic compound (0.5 g), solid potassium hydroxide (2 g) and 5 drops of water in a nickel crucible for about 10 minutes with occasional stirring. Acidify the solution with dilute sulphuric acid.. Evolution of sulphur dioxide gas indicates the presence of sulphuric group. Sulphur dioxide may be detected by means of a filter paper moistened with acidified potassium dichromate solution which turns the paper green.

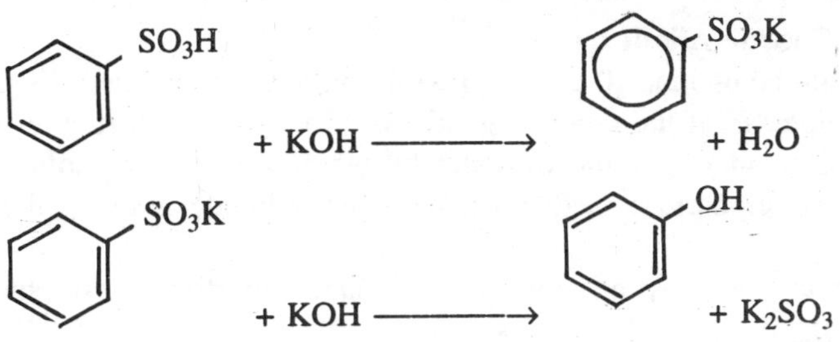

$$K_2SO_3 + H_2SO_4 \longrightarrow K_2SO_4 + H_2O + SO_2$$

(b) Thiourea $(\text{—NH}-\overset{\overset{S}{\|}}{C}-\text{NH}-)$

(i) Heat an organic compound (100 mg) with sodium hydroxide solution (2 ml) for about 1 minute. Cool down the solution and add 2 drops of aqueous lead acetate. Appearance of a dark brown or black colour indicates the presence of thiourea due to formation of sulphide.

$$R-NH-\overset{\overset{S}{\|}}{C}-NHR + 4NaOH \longrightarrow 2RNH_2 + Na_2CO_3 + Na_2S + H_2O$$

$$Na_2S + (CH_3COO)_2 Pb \longrightarrow \underset{\text{Lead sulphide}}{PbS} + 2CH_3COONa$$

(ii) Warm a small amount of organic compound with alcoholic solution of yellow mercuric oxide in a test tube. Appearance of black precipitate of mercuric sulphide indicates the presence of thiourea.

$$R\,NH-\underset{\underset{S}{\|}}{C}-NH\,R + HgO \longrightarrow RNH-\overset{\overset{S}{\|}}{C}-NH\,R + \underset{\text{Mercuric sulphide}}{HgS\downarrow}$$

(iii) Melt a small amount of organic compound in a test tube, cool and dissolve the products in water. Add aqueous ferric chloride solution. Appearance of red colour confirms the presence of thiourea.

$$S=C \xrightarrow{\Delta} CNS^-$$

$$FeCl_3 + 3CNS^- \longrightarrow \underset{\substack{\text{Ferric thiocyanate}\\ \text{(Blood red colour)}}}{Fe(CNS)_3} + 3Cl^-$$

(C) Mercaptans (Thiols)

Mercaptans RSH (also thioether or sulphide $R_1—S—R_2$ and disulphides, $R_1—S—S—R_2$), are generally liquid's and have an unplcasant odour.

Alkyl mercaptans are partly soluble in solution of caustic alkalies. Thiophenols are soluble in an alkali hydroxide solution.

Fusion with Caustic Alkali :

Mix the organic compound (0.5 to 1 g) with potassium hydroxide. (3 g) and 4-5 drops of water in nickel crucible. Heat the crucilbe gently with occasional stirring. Allow to cool and dissolve the solid mass in small amount of water by warming. Pour the solution in a test late and add cautiously 50% sulphuric acid (2 ml); hydrogen sulphide is evolved (detected by lead acetate paper).

This test is given by all organic compounds of divalent sulphur (RSH, R_1—S—R and R_1—SS— R_2).

6. Determination of melting point/boiling point — See chapter 9.

7. Confirmatory Test of the Inferred Some Organic Compound

After determining the functional groups and melting point/boiling point, one or two possible organic compounds are selected and specific confirmatory tests for these organic compounds are carried out.

Carboxylic Acids

Aliphatic carboxylic acid

(i) Formic Acid : [HCOOH] [b.p. 100°]

(a) When formic acid is warmed with concentrated sulphuric acid, carbon monoxide gas is evolved which burns with blue flame.

(b) Formic acid decolourizes acidic permanganate solution.

(c) It gives red colour with ferric chloride.

(d) To the formic acid (1 ml) in a test tube, add a little sodium hydrogen sulphate, warm and then add sodium nitroprusside solution; a greenish blue colour is obtained.

(e) Formic acid gives white precipitate with mercuric chloride solution.

(ii) Acetic Acid : [CH_3 COOH] [B.P 118°]

(a) To acetic acid (1 ml) acid, add 10 drops of absolute ethyl alcohol and 10 drops of concentrated sulphuric acid. Heat gently for 5 minutes, cool and pour into water (5 ml) in a dish; a pleasant fruity smell of ethyl acetate is obtained.

(b) It gives red colour with $FeCl_3$ solution.

(c) It does not decolourizes potassium permanganate solution.

(iii) Oxalic Acid : [$(COOH)_2$] [m.p. 118°]

(a) Take the aqueous solution of oxalic acid (2 ml), add glacial acetic acid (1 ml) and 2-3 drops of aqueous calcium chloride solution; white precipitate, insoluble in acetic acid but soluble in dilute hydrochloric acid is obtained.

(b) Add 5 drops of concentrated sulphuric acid to a small amount of the compound in a dry test tube. Warm the contents gently by rotating the end of the tube over a small flame and turn the mouth of the tube periodically to the flame; characteristic blue flame of carbon monoxide appears.

(c) Heat the aqueous solution of the compound with acidic potassium permanganate solution; purple colour of the solution is discharged.

(iv) Succinic Acid : [COOH—CH_2—CH_2—COOH], [m.p. 185°C]

(a) To a small amount of the acid in a test tube, add a pinch of zinc dust and ammonium hydroxide. Heat the mixture and then place a match stick soaked in concentrated hydrochloric acid in the vapours coming out of the tube which becomes red in colour.

(b) In a test tube, take the neutral solution of the acid (2 ml), add calcium chloride solution

(2 ml), shake and boil for 2 minutes. On scratching the sides of test tube, a white precipitate of calcium succinate, soluble in acetic acid, is obtained.

(c) Add dilute hydrochloric acid to an aqueous solution of the acid. Now add neutral aqueous ferric chloride solution, buff precipitate is obtained.

(d) In a test tube, take the acid (2 g) and twice its amount of resorinol and add concentrated sulphuric acid (1 ml). Heat until the mixture becomes dark brown, look and then pour it in a beaker containing water made alkaline with sodium hydroxide solution, an orange green flourescence is obtained.

Aromatic Carboxylic Acids

(v) Benzoic Acid : C_6H_5COOH [m.p. 121°]

(a) To the acid (0.2 g) in a test tube, add the nitrating mixture (2 ml) (equal amounts of concentrated nitric and concentrated sulphuric acid). Heat carefully for 5-10 minute, cool and pour in a beaker containing water, a pale yellow solid separates out.

(b) When benzoic acid is heated with sodalime, vapours of benzene are evolved.

(vi) Phthalic Acid : [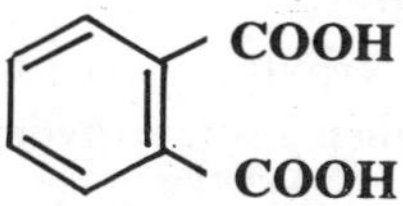] (m.p. 195°)

(a) Mix a rice grain of the substance with the double amount of phenol in a dry test tube. Add 2 drops of concentrated sulphuric acid and heat gently till the mixture attains red-brown colour. Cool, add few drops of water followed by gradual addition of aqueous sodium hydroxide solution with shaking till the solution becomes alkaline; red colour is produced due to formation of phenophthalein; the colour is discharged on adding an acid.

(b) Mix a rice grain of the substance with the double amount of resorcinol. Add 2 drops of concentrated sulphuric and heat gently till the mixture attains red brown colour. Cool, add few drops of water and then aqueous sodium hydroxide till the solution becomes alkaline. Take out this alkaline solution (1 ml) in another test tube and fill up the latter with water; yellow green fluorescence appears.

(vii) Cinnamic Acid 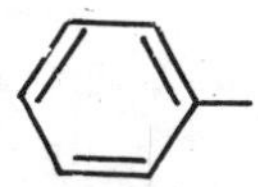 **— CH = CH . COOH** [m.p. 178°]

(a) Add a pinch of compound to a solution of potassium permanganate, the pink colour is discharged and a brown precipitate is produced accompanied by bitter almond smell of benzaldehyde.

(b) Add concentrated sulphuric acid to the compound, heat gently; a green colouration changing to brownish red is produced.

(c) To the neutral solution, add ferric chloride, a light yellow precipitate is produced.

Hydroxy Carboxylic Acids

(i) Lactic Acid : [$CH_3CHOH\ COOH$] [m.p. 18°]

(a) Take acidic solution, add concentrated sulphuric acid and warm; brisk effervescence of carbon dioxide, sulphur dioxide and carbon monoxide appears.

(b) Warm a drop of the acid solution with concentrated sulphuric acid (2 ml) till the solution becomes pale yellow. Cool and add 2 drops of 5% guaiacol solution in alcohol; intense red colour is developed.

(c) It decolourizes acidic potassium permanganate solution on warming.

(d) It gives iodoform test.

(ii) Citric Acid : (HOOCCH$_2$. C (OH) COOH. CH$_2$ COOH. H$_2$O) [m.p. 100°]

(a) To the neutral solution (2 ml) of the acid, add aqueous calcium chloride solution (2 ml). No precipitate is obtained in cold but on heating white shining crystals of calcium citrate separate out.

(b) To the aqueous solution (2 ml) of the acid, add Deniges reagent (1 ml) (mercuric oxide in sulphuric acid), boil and add potassium permanganate solution drop by drop. The purple colour disappears and a white precipitate is obtained.

(c) Take a mixture of small amount of acid and β-naphthol in a dry test-tube and add concentrated sulphuric acid; a blue colour confirms the presence of citric acid.

(d) To aqueous solution of the acid, few drops of silver nitrate solution are added. A white precipitate of silver citrate is obtained. Dissolve the precipitate in ammonium hydroxide. On standing the test tube in boiling water, silver deposits on the walls of test tube.

(iii) Tartaric Acid : [HOOC. CH (OH). COOH] [m.p. 169°]

(a) It reduces ammonical silver nitrate solution.

(b) To acid solution in water, add one drop of ferrous sulphate solution, shake and add one drop of hydrogen peroxide solution and then sodium hydroxide solution (2 ml). An intense violet colour appears.

(c) To the acid solution, add cobalt nitrate solution followed by excess of sodium hydroxide solution. It shows no colour in cold, blue colour on warming, again colourless on cooling.

(d) It gives green colour with β-naphthol in concentrated sulphuric acid. The colour changes to orange on dilution.

(e) Take the neutral solution (3 ml) of the acid, add aqueous calcium chloride solution (1 ml) and shake vigrously. A heavy, white crystalline precipitate, soluble on boiling with glacial acetic acid (1 ml) appears.

(f) Heat the acid, (0.2 g), resorcinol (0.2 g) and concentrated sulphuric acid (2 ml) in a test tube. Violet colour appears.

(g) To the aqueous solution, add 5% solution of ammonium vanadate, acidify it with dilute acetic acid; orange colour appears.

Alcohols

Aliphatic Alcohols

(i) Methyl Alcohol : [CH$_3$ OH] [b.p. 65°]

(a) Heat a copper wire to redness and dip it in the alcohol (2 ml) taken in a test tube. Pungent smell of formaldehyde is produced.

(b) In a dry test tube, take the substance (1 ml), a pinch of salicylic acid and 5-6 drops of concentrated sulphuric acid.. Heat the reaction mixture for 2 minutes, cool and pour in excess amount of water. A characteristic smell of oil of winter green is produced.

(c) On adding potassium dichromate and sulphuric acid to the substance in cold, formaldehyde is formed. The resultant solution, when warmed with a pinch of orcinol, gives a precipitate which is dissolved in sodium hydroxide with green fluorescence.

(ii) Ethyl Alcohol : [C$_2$ H$_5$ OH] [b.p. 78°]

(a) To the substance (2 ml) in a test tube, add glacial acetic acid (2 ml) and concentrated sulphuric acid (1 ml). On heating a fruity smell of ethyl acetate is produced.

(b) **Iodoform Test :** On addition of 3-4 drops of iodine solution and then sodium hydroxide solution drop by drop to the substance and warming, the brown colour of Iodine disappears and yellow precipitate of iodoform having characteristic smell is formed.

(iii) Glycerol : [CH_2OH CHOH CH_2 OH] [b.p. 290°]

(a) To a small amount of the substance, add a pinch of $KHSO_4$. On heating, an irritating pungent smell of acrolein is observed.

(b) It reduces Tollen's reagent (ammonical silver nitrate solution).

(c) To equal amount of substance and phenol in a test tube, add few drops of concentrated sulphuric acid and heat to 130°. Cool, add 10 water (10 ml) and ammonia solution; a red colour is produced. The colour reappears on warming the mixture and again vanishes on cooling.

(d) To borax solution (5 ml), add a drop of phenolphthalein solution when a pink colour is obtained. On addition of 2 or 3 drops of the substance and shaking, the pink colour disappears.

Aromatic Alcohols

(iv) Benzyl Alcohol : [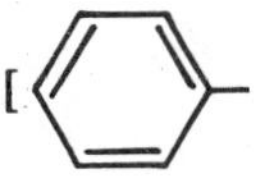 CH_2OH] [b.p. 205°]

(a) To dilute nitric acid (2 ml) in a test tube, add 1-2 drops of substance and keep the tube in boiling water for 2 minutes. Pale yellow emulsion along with strong bitter almond smell is produced due to formation of benzaldehyde.

(b) On oxidation with potassium permanganate in aqueous solution, it yields benzoic acid, m.p. 121°C.

(c) To the substance (1 ml) in a test tube, add concentrated hydrochloric acid (1 ml), shake and stand the tube in boiling water. The mixture becomes clear initially but within a minute white emulsion appears due to formation of benzyl chloride. On keeping the contents undisturbed benzyl chloride forms, separated as colourless upper layer.

(IV) Phenols

(i) Phenol : [C_6H_5OH] [m.p. 42°]

(a) It gives violet colour with ferric chloride.

(b) Heat a mixture of phenol and phthalic acid (2 : 1) after adding few drops of concentrated sulphuric acid. Pour few drops of the resultant product into a beaker containing dilute solution of sodium hydroxide. A pink red colour is obtained due to formation of phenolphthalein.

(c) To small amount of phenol, add hot fuming nitric acid. Heat and then pour the contents in water; a pale yellow solid is obtained.

(d) **Liebermann's Test :** To a small amount of the substance in a test tube, add few crystals of solid sodium nitrite and then few drops of concentrated sulphuric acid; a green or blue colour is obtained which changes to red on dilution and again turns blue green on making the solution alkaline with sodium hydroxide solution.

(ii) Resorcinol : [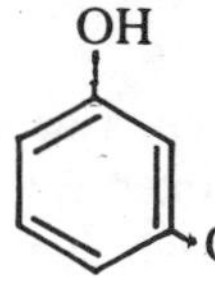 OH] [m.p. 110°]

(a) It gives blue violet colour with neutral aqueous ferric chloride solution.

(b) Phthalein Test : In a dry test tube, take the substance and phthalic acid in (2 : 1 ratio) and add concentrated sulphuric acid (2 ml). Heat the contents first gently and then strongly for 5 minute. Then pour the contents of the tube in a beaker containing dilute solution of sodium hydroxide; an intense yellow green fluorescence is produced due to formation of fluorescein.

(c). To small amount of the substance, add 2 drops of chloroform and sodium hydroxide solution (2 ml) and warm; red colour with green fluorescence is obtained.

(d) It does not reduces Fehling's solution or Tollen's reagent.

(iii) o-Cresol : [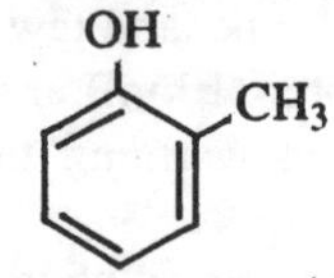] [b.p. 191°]

(a) It responds to Liebermann reaction.

(b) It gives 'Phthalein test' described under phenol.

(c) It gives violet colour with aqueous ferric chloride.

(iv) m - Cresol : [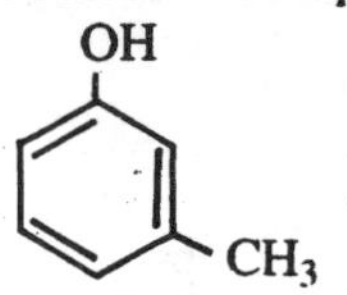] [b.p. 202°]

(a) A mixture of original compound and phthalic anhydride is warmed. On addition of sodium hydroxide solution, a blue violet colour is formed

(b) It gives blue violet colour with ferric chloride solution.

(c) It responds positively to Liebermann reaction.

(d) It gives 'Phthalein test' as described under phenol but instead of pink colour a blue - violet colour is obtained.

(v) p-Cresol : [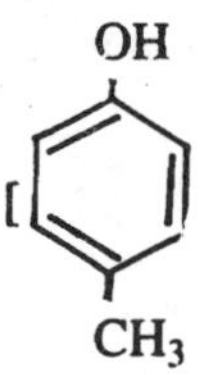] [b.p. 202°]

(a) Take a small amount of the substance in a dry test tube. Add to it few crystals of sodium nitrite and then few drops of concentrated sulphuric acid. Shake the test tube thoroughly; red colour appears.

(b) It gives blue colour with ferric chloride in water.

(vi) α-Naphthol : [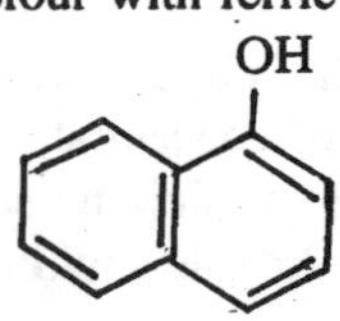] [m.p. 92°]

(a) It does not give colour with neutral aqueous ferric chloride but gives white precipitate.

(b) It gives green colour with titanic acid and concentrated sulphuric acid.

(c) Shake a small amount of the compound with a mixture having equal volume of iodine and potassium iodide and add excess of sodium hydroxide; violet colour appears which rapidly darken followed by a precipitate formation.

(d) Take a small amount of the compound in a test tube and add to it aqueous sodium hydroxide solution (2 ml) and one drop of chloroform; a blue colour appears on warming.

(e) To a small amount of compound in a test tube, add sodium hydroxide solution (2 ml), a drop of carbon tetrachloride and a pinch of copper powder and warm the contents. Blue colour is formed.

(vii) β-Naphthol : [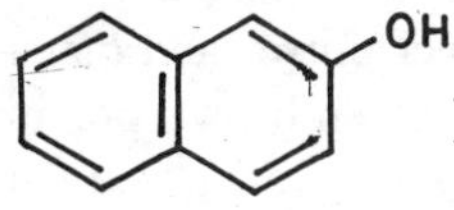] [m.p. 122°]

(a) It does not give colour with neutral ferric chloride solution.
(b) With titanic acid in concentrated sulphuric acid, it gives red colour.
(c) A mixture of the substance, sodium hydroxide and chloroform is warmed. A blue colour is formed.
(d) It gives yellow colour with sodium hypobromite solution (NaOBr).

(viii) Catechol : [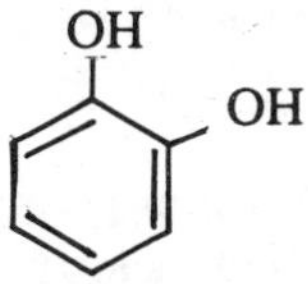] m.p. 104°]

(a) It gives green colour with ferric chloride in aqueous solution. On addition of ammonia the colour changes to deep red.
(b) Solution of substance in sodium hydroxide turns brown on standing in air.
(c) It reduces Fehling's solution and Tollen's reagent
(d) To the aqueous solution (2 ml), add lead acetate solution (2 ml); a white precipitate is formed immediately.

(ix) Quinol : [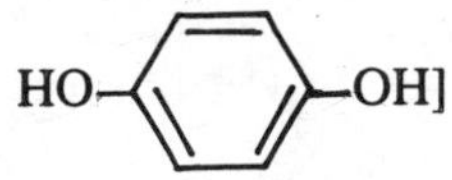] [m.p. 172°]

(a) It reduces ammonical silver nitrate solution in cold.
(b) Its aqueous solution gives brown colour on shaking with sodium hydroxide solution.
(c) Shake aqueous solution with ferric chloride solution.
A blue colour appears which immediately changes to reddish brown.

(V) Aldehydes

Aliphatic Aldehydes

(i) Formaldehyde : [HCHO] [b.p. 97-98°]

(a) It gives reddish brown precipitate (charging to yellow green) with dilute solution of Nesseler's reagent
(b) On evaporation, a white residue of paraformaldehyde is obtained.
(c) To aqueous solution of the substance (2 ml) in a test tube, add few crystals of resorcinol and then pour concentrated sulphuric acid (2 ml) carefully from side of the test tube. A red ring is formed at the junction of liquids and a white precipitate appears in the aqueous layer which turns violet red.

(ii) Acetaldehyde : [CH_3CHO] [b.p. 210°]

(a) To the aqueous solution of the substance (2 ml), add aqueous sodium nitroprusside solution (2 ml) and 5 drops of sodium hydroxide solution. A deep wine-red colour is produced

(b) On adding a few drop of aqueous solution of the substance to dilute solution of benzidine hydrochloride, a yellow colour is produced.

(c) It reduces Tollen's reagent to yield a silver mirror and black precipitate.

(d) It reduces Fehling's solution to yield a reddish brown precipitate of cuprous oxide.

(e) A very dilute aqueous solution gives a light yellow precipitate with Nesseler's solution while concentrated solution gives a red precipitate turning grey.

(f) To aqueous solution of the substance (2 ml), add 20% potassium hydroxide solution (2 ml) and boil for 1 minute; the solution becomes yellow and finally a yellow precipitate changing to orange with a disagreeable smell is obtained.

Aromatic aldehyde

(iii) Benzaldehyde : [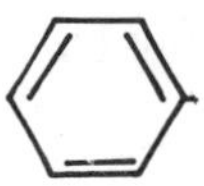 CHO] [b.p. 179°]

(a) To the substance in a test tube, add alkaline potassium permanganate solution (2 ml) and heat the contents for 5 minutes. Filter and acidify the filtrate with dilute hydrochloric acid; a white precipitate of benzoic acid is obtained.

(b) It does not reduce Fehling's solution.

(c) Take the substance (1 ml), 5 drops of acetone, ethyl alcohol (5 ml) and dilute sodium hydroxide (2 ml) in a boiling tube and boil the contents for 2 minute. Cool, shake vigorously and add water (20 ml). A yellow solid, dibenzyl acetone, separates out.

(d) To the substance (1 ml), add dimethylaniline (1 ml) and small amount of fused zinc chloride. Heat the mixture; a dark green precipitate of benzaldimethylaniline is produced.

(VI) Ketones

Aliphatic Ketone

(i) Acetone : [CH_3COCH_3] [b.p. 56°]

(a) **Iodoform Test :** Add 3-4 drops of iodine solution and then aqueous sodium hydroxide drop by drop to the substance and warm. The brown colour of iodine disappears and a yellow precipitate of iodoform having characteristic smell is formed.

(b) Dissolve a small amount of o-nitrobenazaldehyde in original substance (2 ml) and pour in a beaker containing alkaline water. A blue colour due to formation of indigo is produced.

(c) To saturated solution of sodium bisulphite (2 ml), add few drops of substance; white crystals of bisulphite adduct are formed with evolution of heat.

Aromatic ketones

(ii) Acetophenone : [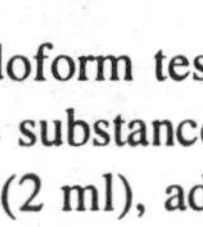 —CO—CH_3] [b.p. 202°]

(a) It responds to iodoform test described under acetone.

(b) On dissolving the substance in concentrated sulphuric acid, orange colour is produced.

(c) To the substance (2 ml), add alkaline potassium permanganate solution (2 ml) and heat for 5 minute. Cool, filter and acidify the filtrate with dilute hydrochloric acid; a white precipitate of benzoic acid is obtained.

(d) Its aqueous solution gives wine red colour with alkaline sodium nitroprusside solution; on addition of acetic acid, the colour changes to blue.

(iii) Benzophenone : $[C_6H_5COC_6H_5]$ [m.p. 49°]

(a) When the substances is dissolved in concentrated sulphuric acid, a yellow solution is obtained.

(b) Fusion of the substance with sodium produces deep blue colour.

Esters

Aliphatic ester

(i) Ethyl Acetate : $[CH_3COOC_2H_5]$ [b.p. 77°]

(a) It is colourless liquid with an apple like odour.

(b) It is slightly soluble in water.

Aromatic ester

(ii) Methyl Benzoate : $[C_6H_5COOCH_3]$ [b.p. 199°]

(a) It is an aromatic, colourless liquid.

(b) The compound is heated with 10% aqueous sodium hydroxide solution, precipitate of benzoic acid is obtained. It is filtered, washed with cold water and dried, m.p. 122°.

(iii) Ethyl Benzoate $[C_6H_5COOC_2H_5]$ [b.p. 213°]

(a) Boil the ester with sodium hydroxide solution for few minutes. Cool and add ferric chloride solution; a buff coloured precipitate is formed.

Carbohydrates

(i) Glucose : $[CH_2OH(CHOH)_4CHO]$ [m.p. 80° (hydrate)]

(a) It reduces Fehling's solution, Tollen's reagent and Barfoed's reagent

(b) Add lead acetate (1 g) to aqueous solution (2 ml) of the substance, boil and add dilute ammonia solution (5 ml). Continue boiling for 5 minutes. A rose pink colour confirms the presence of glucose.

(c) It reduces Benedict's solution (solution of copper sulphate, sodium citrate and sodium carbonate) to yield yellow orange or orange red precipitate.

(ii) Fructose : $[CH_2OH \, . \, [CHOH]_3 \, COCH_2OH]$ [m.p. 95-105°]

(a) It reduces Fehling's solution and Tollen's reagent.

(b) It gives blue colour on warning with ammonium molylbdate solution.

(c) To a small amount of the compound, add equal amount of resorcinol and concentrated hydrochloric acid (1 ml). A red colour is obtained on warming the mixture.

(d) It reduces Barfoed's reagent (cupric acetate in acetic acid) on warming.

(e) It gives rapid furfural test.

(f) Take a small amount of the compound in a test tube, add to it half the amount of sodium or selenium dioxide and dilute hydrochloric acid (2 ml). Heat the test tube in boiling water bath for 2 minute. A finely divided red precipitate of selenium is obtained.

(iii) Sucrose : $[C_{12}H_{22}O_{11}]$ [m.p. 185°]

(a) It does not react with Fehling's solution or with phenylhydrazine. However, after hydrolysis, by warming with dilute HCl, it reduces Fehling's solution and reacts with phenyl-hydrazine.

(b) On treatment with concentrated sulphuric acid, it is charred in cold.

(c) It gives red colour on boiling with saturated ammonical nickle sulphate solution and then adding dilute sulphuric acid.

(d) On warming with cobalt nitrate and sodium hydroxide solution, a violet colour is produced.
(e) To aqueous solution of the substance (2 ml), add a pinch of resorcinol and concentrated hydrochloric acid (2 ml). Boil for 2 minute. A deep wine red colour is produced.
(f) Blue solution is formed with copper sulphate and sodium hydroxide solution.

Amine

Aromatic amine

(i) Aniline : [$C_6H_5NH_2$] [b.p. 183°]

(a) With bleaching powder, it gives purple colour.
(b) On warming with alcoholic potassium hydroxide and chloroform, an unpleasant odour of phenylisocynate is produced.
(c) Dissolve a drop of the compound in ether (2 ml) and to it add water (10 ml). Add dilute solution (1 ml) of bleaching powder and shake. A purple colour is obtained.
(d) Dissolve small amount of potassium dichromate in concentrated sulphuric acid and to this add 1 drop of the substance. A blue or black colour is obtained.

(ii) Benzylamine : [$C_6H_5CH_2NH_2$] [b.p. 185°]

(a) On oxidation with alkaline potassium permanganate, it yields benzoic acid, m.p. 121°.
(b) It is miscible with water.

(iii) Diphenylamine : [$(C_6H_5)_2$ NH] [m.p. 54°]

(a) To the solution of the compound in concentrated sulphuric acid, add one drop of aqueous sodium nitrite solution. A deep blue colour is produced.
(b) The solution of the amine in concentrated hydrochloric acid with a trace of nitric acid forms blue colour.

(iv) Dimethylaniline : [$C_6H_5N(CH_3)_2$] [b.p. 193°]

(a) To the substance (1 ml), add 0.5 g of oxalic acid dissolved in alcohol (5 ml). A white precipitate of oxalate of dimethyl aniline is obtained.

Nitro Compounds

(i) Nitrobenzene : [$C_6H_5NO_2$] [b.p. 210°]

(a) To the substances (1 ml) in a boiling tube add few pieces of tin (or a pinch of zinc dust or tin chloride) and concentrated hydrochloric acid (2 ml). Boil the mixture for 5 minute; aniline is produced. It is filtered and the filtrate divided into 2 parts.
In the first part perform dye test; positive result is obtained.
In the second part perform carbylamine test; positive result is obtained.
(b) To a few drops of the substance, add a pinch of zinc dust, glacial acetic acid (2 ml) and boil. Add water (2 ml) and then a solution of sodium hydroxide drop by drop till the mixture is alkaline. Add 2 drops of this resultant solution to sodium hypochlorite solution (5 ml). Violet colour is produced.

(ii) m - Dinitrobenzene : [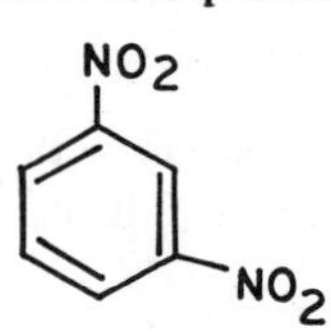] [m.p. 90°]

(a) It gives red-brown colour on boiling with sodium hydroxide solution.
(b) Dissolve a pinch of the compound in acetone (2 ml) and add a drop of sodium hydroxide

solution. A violet blue colour is produced which changes to violet red on adding acetic acid.

(c) Dissolve a pinch of substance in dilute sodium hydroxide and boil. To this, add a very small amount of glucose (or tin chloride). Violet colour is produced.

(iii) o-Toluidine 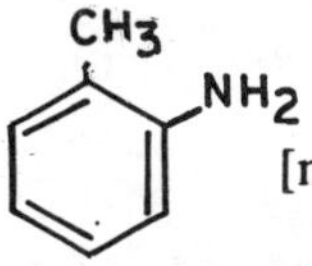 [m.p. 200°]

(a) Shake its ethereal solution with bleaching powder solution or sodium hypochlorite solution. The ethereal layer becomes brown.

(b) Add 2-3 drops of the compound to potassium dichromate solution. A blue colour is produced which changes to green on dilution.

(iv) p-Toluidine 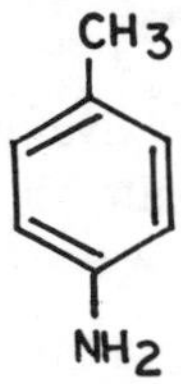 [m.p. 45°]

(a) Dissolve the compound in 50% sulphuric acid and divide into two portion.

(i) To one portion add nitric acid. A blue colour is formed which changes gradually to violet red and then brown.

(ii) To another portion, add potassium dichromate solution. A yellow colour is produced.

(b) Take a pinch of the compound in water (5 ml). Add 2-3 ml of concentrated hydrochloric acid, ferric chloride solution (1 ml) and heat the mixture. An orange reddish colour is produced.

Aliphatic Amides

(i) Acetamide : [CH_3CONH_2] [m.p. 82°]

(a) On heating the substance with concentrated sulphuric acid, a strong smell of vinegar is produced due to formation of acetic acid.

(b) When the compound is heated with aniline, it yields acetanilide, m.p 114°, with evolution of ammonia.

(ii) Urea : [H_2NCONH_2] [m.p. 132°]

(a) Biuret test : Heat a small amount of the substance in a dry test tube. The solid melts and ammonia is evolved. Cool the tube when a white residue is left in it. Dissolve it in water (2 ml), add a drop of copper sulphate solution and sodium hydroxide solution (2 ml) when violet colour is produced.

(b) Dissolve a small amount of the substance in dilute hydrochloric acid, cool and add few drops of sodium nitrite solution to it. Nitrogen gas is evolved with effervescence.

(c) Add 2 or 3 ml of concentrated nitric acid to the substance (0.5 g) and boil. On cooling white crystals of urea nitrate are obtained.

Aromatic Amide

(iii) Benzamide : [$C_6H_5CONH_2$] [m.p. 129°]

(a) Boil a small amount of the substance with dilute sodium hydroxide for 5 minute, cool and acidify with dilute hydrochloric acid; a white precipitate of benzoic acid, m.p 121°, is obtained.

(b) Mix a small amount of the substance with either sodalime or phosphorus pentachloride in a dry ignition tube and heat; smell of bitter almonds is produced due to formation of benzonitrile.

Aliphatic Anilide

(i) Acetanilide : [$C_6H_5NHCOCH_3$] [m.p. 114°]

(a) With concentrated nitric and sulphuric acids, it yields p-nitro derivative, m.p. 216°; on ignition.

(b) On bromination with bromine in acetic acid, it yields p-bromo derivative, m.p 167°.

Aromatic Anilide

(ii) Benzanilide : [$C_6H_5NHCOC_6H_5$] [m.p. 161°]

(a) With bromine in acetic acid, it yields p-bromo derivative m.p 204°.

(b) On nitration in cold, it yield a mixture of o-nitro derivative, m.p 94°, and p-nitro derivative, m.p 199°.

Halogen Compound

(i) Chloroform : [$CHCl_3$] [b.p. 61°]

(a) To a small amount of the substance, add few crystals of resorcinol and aqueous sodium hydroxide (2 ml) and boil; red colour is produced.

(b) **Carbylamine Test :** To the substance (1 ml), add aniline (1 ml) and potassium hydroxide (4 ml). Boil for 2 minutes. Highly offensive odour of phenyl isocyanide is observed.

(c) Boil a few drop of the substance with pyridine and sodium hydroxide solution and allow to stand, pyridine layer becomes red.

(ii) Iodoform : [CHI_3] [m.p. 119°]

(a) On heating the substance, violet vapours of iodine are produced.

(b) To a small amount of substance, add resorcinol (1 g) and alcoholic sodium hydroxide solution (2 ml) and warm. A red colour changing to violet is produced.

(c) To the 20 % sodium hydroxide solution (5 ml), add a pinch of substance and 4-5 drops of pyridine. Boil and allow to stand when pyridine layer becomes red in colour.

(iii) Carbon Tetrachloride : [CCl_4] [b.p. 78°]

(a) **Carbylamine Test :** To 2-3 drops of the substance, add 2-3 drops of aniline and alcoholic potassium hydroxide solution (2 ml) and boil for 5 minute. An obnoxious smell of phenyl isocyanide is produced but more slowly then chloroform.

(b) If the compound is first reduced to chloroform by adding a pinch of zinc dust, 1 ml dilute hydrochloric acid (1 ml) and boiling , then it responds to carbylamine reaction.

(iv) Chlorobenzene : 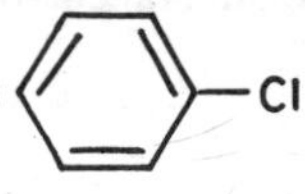 [b.p. 132°]

(a) It is an aromatic, colourless liquid with pleasant almond like odour, non-miscible with water.

(b) It is inflammable.

Sulphonic Acids

(i) Benzene Sulphonic Acid : 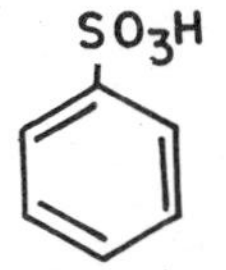 [m.p. 65°]

It is freely soluble in water and alcohol; slightly soluble in benzene, insoluble in ether and carbon disulphide.

Derivatives : (a) Amide, m.p 153°, (b) Anilide, m.p. 110°,
(c) S—Benzyl iso-thiuronium salt, m.p.148°

(ii) p-Toluene Sulphonic Acid: 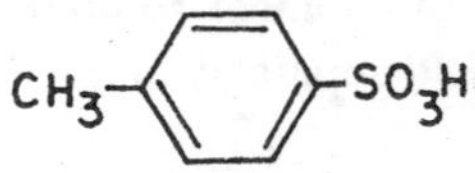 [m.p. 92°]

It is soluble in dilute NaOH, alcohol and ether.

Derivatives : (a) Amide, m.p. 137°, (b) Anilide, m.p 103°, (c) Chloride, m.p. 69°

(iii) Sulphanilic Acid : $H_2N—OSO_3H$ [m.p. 288°] 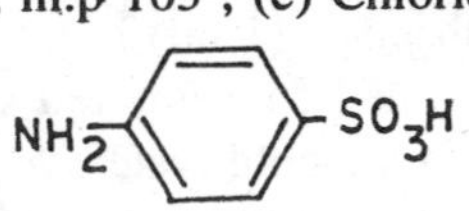

(a) When heated with sodalime, it forms aniline, b.p 183°.
(b) To a solution of $NaHCO_3$, add a pinch of substance. Carbon dioxide gas is evolved with effervescence.
(c) On diazotization and then coupling with alkaline β-naphthnol, an orange-red dye is produced.
(d) When oxidized with potassium dichromate and concentrated sulphuric acid, it forms p-benzoquinone having a characteristic pungent odour.

Thioureas

(i) Thiourea: $[H_2NCSNH_2]$ [m.p. 180°]

(a) Boil a small amount of the substance with sodium hydroxide. Ammonia gas is evolved. To the solution, add water (5 ml) and a drop of ferric chloride. A blood red colour is produced due to formation of ferric thiocyanate.
(b) Dissolve a small amount of the compound by heating in dilute acetic acid (2 ml). To the hot solution, add potassium ferrocyanide solution (2 ml). A green colour changing to blue appears.
(c) The compound dissolved in sodium hydroxide solution gives black precipitate with lead acetate.
(d) Heat a small amount of the compound over a flame until the solid melts, dissolve the residue by shaking with water (2 ml) and then add aqueous ferric chloride (2 ml). Fill the test tube with water and shake. A deep red solution is produced.

(ii) Phenyl thiourea : $[C_6H_5.NH.CS.NH_2]$ [m.p. 154°]

(a) When boiled with sodium hydroxide solution, it gives ammonia.
(b) On boiling with dilute hydrochloric acid, it produces pungent offensive odour of phenyl isocyanide.
(c) Take a small amount of the compound in a dry test tube and add to it 5 drops of concentrated sulphuric acid. Heat for a moment, cool and carefully add water (5 ml). Again cool and then add aqueous sodium nitrite solution (5 ml). Add this solution (2 ml) to alkaline solution of β-naphthol (5 ml). A red solution is formed.
(d) Repeat the above test up to the stage of dilution with water. Now make the solution alkaline by adding sodium hydroxide solution and then hold a strip of moistened red litmus paper near the mouth of the tube. The colour changes to blue.

Hydrocarbons

(i) Benzene : 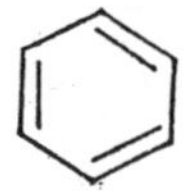 [b.p. 80°]

(a) Take the substance (1 ml) in a boiling tube and to this, add concentrated nitric acid (2 ml) and then concentrated sulphuric acid (2 ml) drop by drop with shaking. Heat the contents for about 30 minutes, cool and pour the reaction mixture in ice-cold water. A yellow oily liquid is solidified on standing.

(b) To the substance (2 ml), add ammonical solution of nickel cyanide (2 ml). A white coloured, violet tinted compound separates out.

(ii) Toluene : 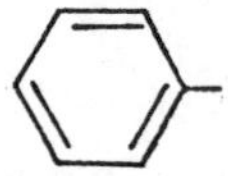 CH_3 [b.p. 110°]

(a) To the substance (1 ml) in a boiling test tube, add nitration mixture concentrated nitric acid (3 ml) and concentrated sulphuric acid (3 ml); Allow the reaction mixture to cool and pour in ice-cold water. A yellow solid of 2, 4, 6-trinitrotoluene separates out.

(b) Heat the substance (1 ml) with a pinch of magnessium oxide and concentrated sulphuric acid (1 ml) in the presence of few crystals of copper sulphate. Benzeldehyde is formed which can be detected due to its bitter almond smell.

(iii) Naphthalene : 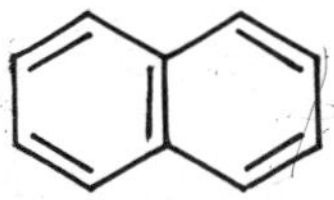 [m.p. 80°]

(a) Dissolve small amount of the substance in chloroform and add dry aluminium chloride. A green colour develops.

(b) Oxidation with concentrated sulphuric acid in the presence of mercuric sulphate yields phthalic acid, m.p 195°.

(iv) Anthracene : 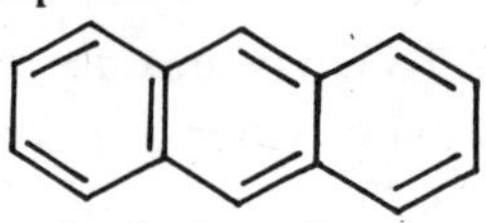 [m.p. 216°]

(a) Prepare a saturated solution of anthracene in xylene and keep it in sunlight for sometime when crystals of dianthracene appears.

(b) Shake a small amount of the substance with saturated solution of picric acid (2 ml) in benzene. A deep red solution is produced.

(c) Heat chromium oxide (1 g) in water (1 ml) and glacial acetic acid (9 ml) in a 100 ml flask until all the chromium oxide has dissolved. Cool, add compound (0.5 g) and boil the contents under reflux gently for 10 minute with occasional shaking. Cool the contents, add water (50 ml), shake and fitter. Wash the anthraquinone with water until it is clear yellow in colour. Test the formation of anthraquinone as described below : Mix two rice grain of the compound with equal amount of zinc dust and add to it aqueous sodium hydroxide solution (5 ml). Boil the contents for about 30 seconds. A deep red colour is produced.

(v) Phenanthrene : 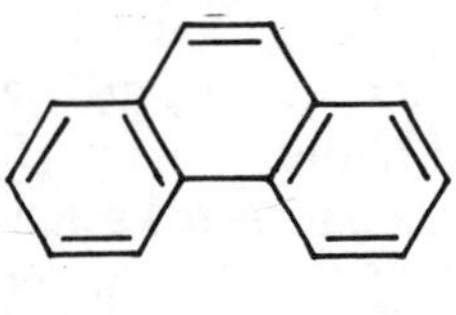 [m.p. 100°]

(a) It dissolves in benzene with light blue fluorescence.

(vi) o-Xylene : 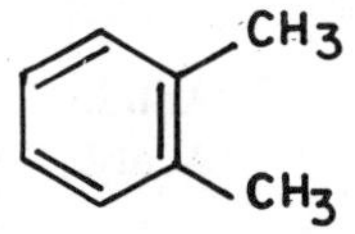 [b.p. 144°]

(a) On oxidation, it produces phthalic acid, m.p 195°.

(vii) m-Xylene : 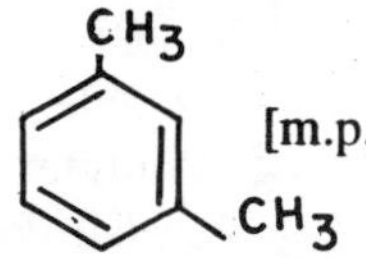 [m.p. 139°]

(a) On warming with a mixture of concentrated nitric and sulphuric acids and pouring the reaction mixture in water, it gives 2, 4, 6-trinitro derivative, m.p 182°.
(b) On oxidation with alkaline potassium permanganate, it yields iosphthalic acid.

(viii) p—Xylene : 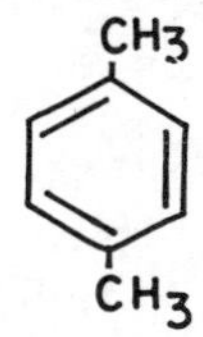 [b.p. 138°]

(a) On oxidation with alkaline potassium permanganate, it yields terephthalic acid.
(b) On warning with a mixture of concentrated sulphuric and nitric acids and pouring the reaction mixture in water, 2, 3, 5-trinitrodervative, m.p 139°, is produced.

Table 10.2. Some Important Organic Compounds with their Common Derivatives

	Compound	*State*	*m.p. or b.p.., °C*	*Derivative, m.p, °C*
Carboxylic Acids				
1.	Formic acid HCOOH	Liquid	b.p. 100°	Amide, 195° Anilide, 47° Ammonium Salt, 114°
2.	Acetic acid CH_3COOH	Liquid	b.p. 118°	Amide, 79° Anilide, 103° Ammonium salt, 66°
3.	Propionic acid CH_3CH_2COOH	Liquid	b.p. 140°	Amide, 82°
4.	Oxalic acid HOOC—COOH	Solid	m.p. 101°	Anilide, 245° Toluidide, 267°
5.	Succinic acid CH_2 COOH | CH_2COOH	Solid	m.p. 185°	Amide, 260° Anilide, 269° Anhydride, 119°
6.	Tartaric acid CHOHCOOH | CHOHCOOH	Solid	m.p.. 170°	Anilide, 126° Toluidide, 264°
7.	Citric acid (hydrated)	Solid	m.p. 100°	Anilide, 115°

No.	Compound	State	Constant	Derivative
	CH_2 COOH | C(OH)COOH | CH_2 COOH			Amide, 210° Acetyl, 175°
8.	Benzoic acid C_6H_5COOH 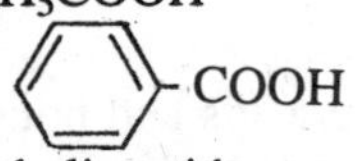	Solid	m.p. 121°	Amide, 108° Anilide, 160° m-Nitrobenzoic acid, 148°
9.	Phthalic acid 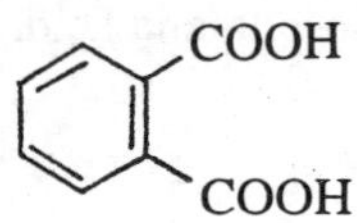	Solid	m.p. 184°	Anhydride, 130° Amide, 220°
10.	Cinnamic acid 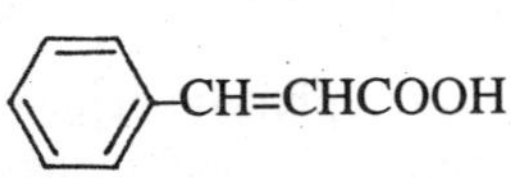	Solid	m.p. 133°	p-Nitro, derivative 285° Anilide, 153° Amide, 141°
11.	Anthranilic acid 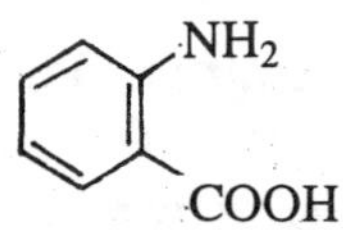	Solid	m.p. 147°	Amide, 108° Anilide, 126° Benzoyl, 182°
12.	Salicylic acid 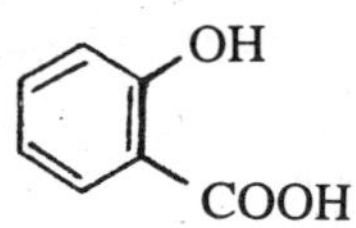	Solid	m.p. 155°	Aspirin, 135° Amide, 139°
13.	Gallic acid	Solid	m.p. 263°	Anilide, 134°
Alcohols				
14.	Methyl alcohol CH_3OH	Liquid	m.p. 65°	3, 5-Dinitrobenzoate, 107°
15.	Ethyl alcohol C_2H_5OH	Liquid	b.p. 70⁰	3,5—Dinitrobenzoate, 94° Iodoform, 119°
16.	n-Propyl alcohol $C_3H_5CH_2OH$	Liquid	b.p. 97°	3,5—Dinitrobenzoate, 75°
17.	n-Butyl alcohol $C_3H_7CH_2OH$	Liquid	b.p. 118°	3, 5-Dinitrobenzoate, 64°
18.	Glycerol	Liquid	b.p. 290°	Tribenzoate, 76°
Phenol				
19.	Phenol 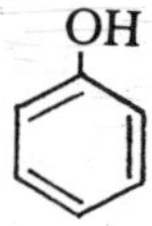	Solid	m.p. 42°	Tribromophenol, 93°

No.	Compound	State	b.p./m.p.	Derivatives
20.	o-Cresol 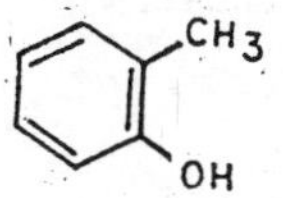	Liquid	b.p. 191°	Bromoderivative, 56° Picrate, 88°
21.	m-Cresol 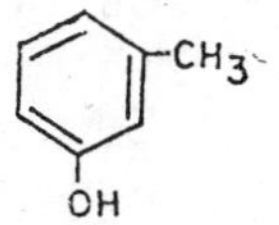	Liquid	b.p. 203°	Bromo derivative, 84° Benzoyl derivative, 54°
22.	p-Cresol 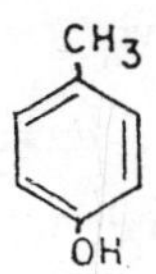	Liquid	b.p. 202°	Benzoyl derivative, 71°
23.	Catechol 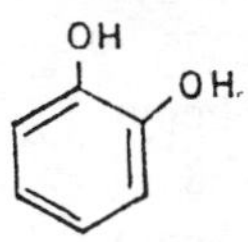	Solid	m.p. 105°	Diacetyl, 123° Dibenzoyl, 199°
24.	Resorcirol 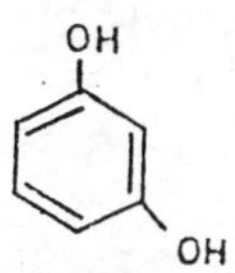	Solid	m.p. 110°	Benzoate, 117° p-Nitrobenzoate, 182° Dibromo, 112°
25.	Pyrogallol 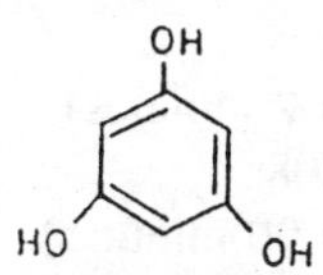	Solid	m.p. 133°	Triacetate, 161°
26.	Hydroquinone 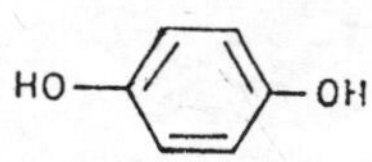	Solid	m.p. 172°	Diacetyl, 123° Dibenzoyl, 199°
27.	α -Naphthol 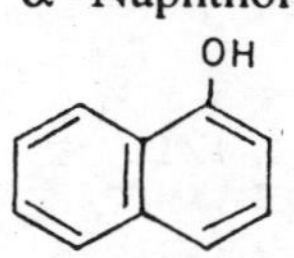	Solid	m.p. 96°	Picrate, 189° Acetyl derivative, 46°
28.	β -Naphthol 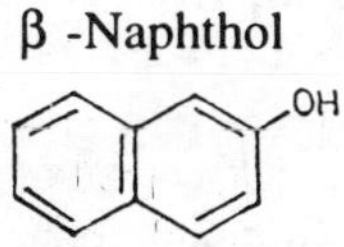	Solid	m.p. 122°	Picrate, 156° Acetyl derivative, 70°

29.	Picric Acid 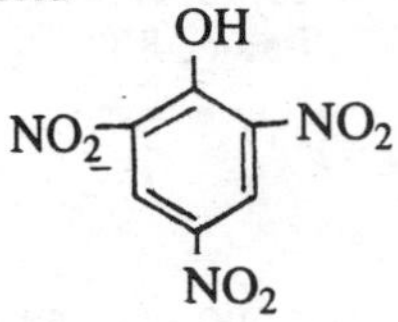	Solid	m.p. 122°	p-Nitrobenzoate, 143° Acetyl derivative, 76°
30.	o-Nitro phenol 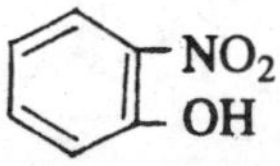	Solid	m.p. 44°	Benzoyl derivative, 142° Picric acid, 122°
Aldehydes and Ketones				
31.	Formaline solution (40% aqueous solution of HCHO)	Liquid	b.p. 98°	2, 4-dinitrophenyl hydrazone, 166°
32.	Acetaldehyde CH_3CHO	Liquid	b.p. 21°	2, 4-Dinitrophenyl hydrazone,168°
33.	Benzaldehyde C_6H_5CHO	Liquid	b.p. 179°	2, 4-Dinitrophenyl hydrazone, 237°
34.	Acetone CH_3COCH_3	Liquid	b.p. 56°	2, 4-Dinitrophenyl hydrazone, 128°
35.	Acetophenone $C_6H_5COCH_3$	Liquid	b.p. 202°	2, 4-Dinitrophenyl hydrazone, 128°
36.	Benzophenone $C_6H_5COC_6H_5$	Solid	m.p. 48°	2, 4-Dinitrophenyl-hydrazone, 229°
Carbohydrates				
37.	D-Glucose ($C_6H_{12}O_6 . H_2O$)	Solid	m.p. 80°	Osazone, 205° (Formed in 5 minutes)
38.	D-Fructose $C_6H_{12}O_6$	Solid	m.p. 95—105°	Osazone, 205° (Formed in 2 minutes)
39.	Lactose (hydrates) $C_{12}H_{22}O_{11}.H_2O$	Solid	m.p. 203°	Osazone, 208° (Formed in 90 minutes)
40.	Sucrose	Solid	m.p. 185°	Octa-acetate, 67°
41.	Starch $(C_6H_{10}O_5)_n$	Solid	Decompose without melting	....
Esters				
42.	Ethyl acetate $CH_3COOC_2H_5$	Liquid	b.p. 77°	Anilide, 115°
43.	Methyl benzoate $C_6H_5COOCH_3$	Liquid	b.p. 213°	Benzoic acid, 121°
44	Ethyl benzoate $C_6H_5COOC_2H_5$	Liquid	b.p. 213°	Benzoic acid, 121°
Hydrocarbons				
45.	Benzene 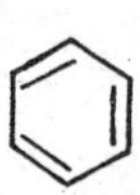	Liquid	b.p. 80°	m—Dinitrotoluene, 90° Picrate, 84°

46.	Toluene $C_6H_5CH_3$	Liquid	b.p. 111°	2,4—Dinitrotoluene, 71°
47.	Diphenyl $C_6H_5 - C_6H_5$	Solid	b.p. 80°	p, p-Dinitro- diphenyl, 234°
48.	Naphthalene 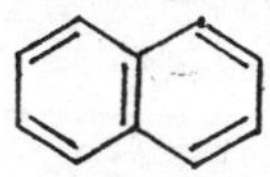	Solid	m.p. 80°	Picrate, 149°
49.	Anthracene 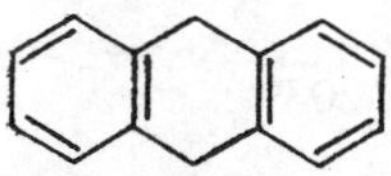	Solid	m.p. 216°	Picrate, 138°
50.	Phenanthrene 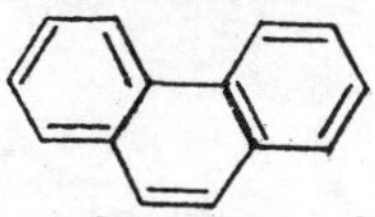	Solid	m.p. 100°	Picrate, 143° 9-Bromophenanthrene, 65°

Amino Compounds

51.	Ethyl amine $C_2H_5NH_2$	Liquid	b.p. 19°	Benzoyl, 71°
52.	Benzyl amine $C_6H_5CH_2NH_2$	Liquid	b.p. 185°	Acetyl, 60° Benzoyl, 105°
53.	Aniline $C_6H_5NH_2$	Liquid	b.p. 183°	Acetyl, 114° Benzoyl, 163°
54.	o–Toluidine 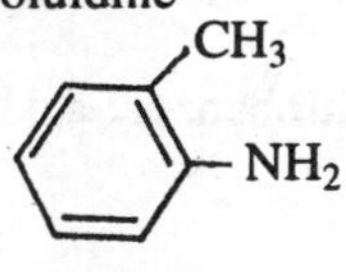	Liquid	b.p. 200°	Acetyl, 112° Benzoyl, 142° Picrate, 214°
55.	m—Toluidine 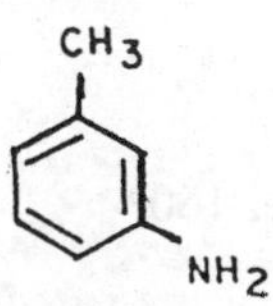	Liquid	b.p. 203°	Acetyl, 65° Benzoyl, 125° Picrates, 195°
56.	p-Toluidine 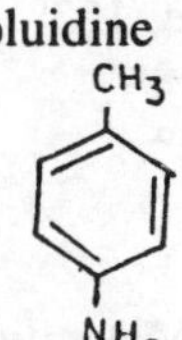	Solid	m.p. 45°	Acetyl, 148° Benzoyl, 158°
57.	α -Naphthylamine 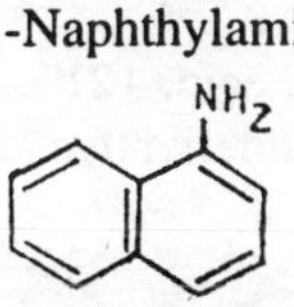	Solid	b.p. 50°	Acetyl, 160° Benzoyl, 161° Picrate, 163°
58.	β-Naphthylamine 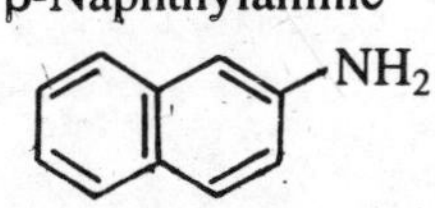	Solid	m.p. 113°	Acetyl, 134° Benzoyl, 162° Picrate, 195°

59. Methyl aniline $C_6H_5NH\text{–}CH_3$	Liquid	b.p. 192°	Acetyl, 103° Benzoyl, 180° Picrate, 182°
60. Diphenylamine $C_6H_5 - NH - C_6H_5$	Solid	m.p. 54°	Acetyl, 103° Benzoyl, 180° Picrate, 182°
61. Dimethylamine $C_6H_5NH(CH_3)_2$	Liquid	b.p. 194°	Picrate, 163°
62. Pyridine C_5H_5N	Liquid	b.p. 115°	Picrate, 167°
63. Quinoline 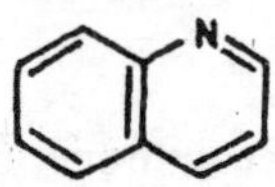	Liquid	b.p. 238°	Picrate, 203°

Nitro Compounds

64. Nitro benzene $C_6H_5NO_2$	Liquid	b.p. 211°	m-Dinitrobenzene, 90°
65. m-Dinitrobenzene 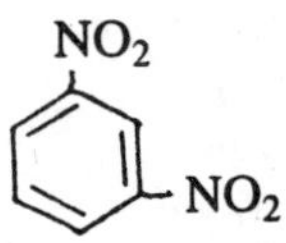	Solid	b.p. 90°	m-Nitroaniline, 114°
66. o-Nitro toluene 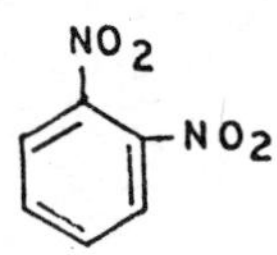	L.iquid	b.p. 220°	2,4-Dinitrotoluene, 70° o-Nitrobenzoic acid, 147°

Amides

67. Acetanide CH_3CONH_2	Solids	m.p. 82°	Anilide, 141°
68. Benzamide $C_6H_5CONH_2$	Solid	m.p. 128°	Anilide, 160°
69. Urea $NH_2CO.NH_2$	Solid	m.p. 132°	Urea nitrate, 163° Anilide, 238° Biuret, 192°

Anilides

70. Acetanilide $CH_3CONH\text{—}O$	Solid	m.p. 114°	p—Bromoacetanilide, 167°
71. Benzanilide 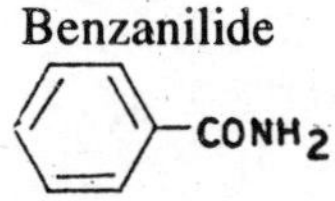	Solid	m.p. 162°	Benzoic acid, 121° p-Bromoderivative, 204°

Compounds having halogens.

(Such compounds are immiscible with water and heavier than it)

72.	Chloroform $CHCl_3$	Liquid	b.p. 61°	——
73.	Iodoform CHI_3	Solid	m.p. 119°	——
74.	Carbon tetrachloride CCl_4	Liquid	b.p. 77°	——
75.	Chlorobenzene C_6H_5Cl	Liquid	b.p. 132°	2, 4-Dinitro derivative, 52°
76.	Bromobenzene C_6H_5Br	Liquid	b.p. 156°	2, 4-Dinitro derivative, 75°
77.	Iodobenzene C_6H_5I	Liquid	b.p. 188°	p-Nitro derivative, 174°
78.	Benzyl Chloride $C_6H_5CH_2Cl$	Liquid	b.p. 179°	p-Nitro derivative, 71°
79.	o-Chlorotoluene	Liquid	b.p. 159°	o-Chlorobenzoic acid, 140°

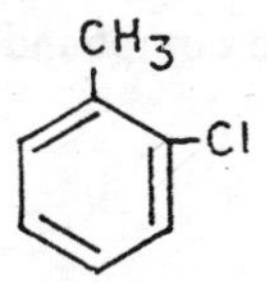

80.	m-Chlorotoluene	Liquid	b.p. 162°	m-Chlorobenzoic acid, 153°

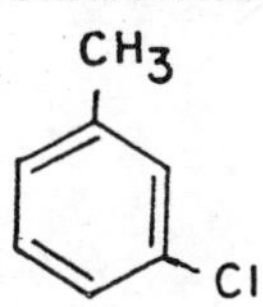

81.	p-Chlorotoluene	Liquid	b.p. 162°	p-Chloro benzoic acid, 162°

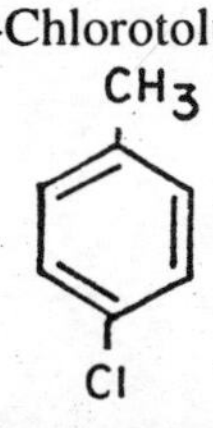

Sulphonic acids

82.	Benzene sulphonic acid $C_6H_5SO_3H$	Solid	m.p. 65°	Amide, 153° Anilide, 110°
83.	p-Toluene sulphonic acid	Solid	m.p. 92°	Anide, 137° Anilide, 103°

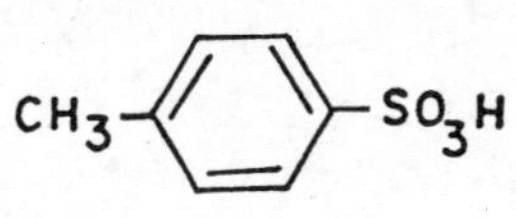

84.	Sulphanilic acid	Solid	m.p. 288°	2,4,6—Tribromo, 119° Sulphonamide, 200°

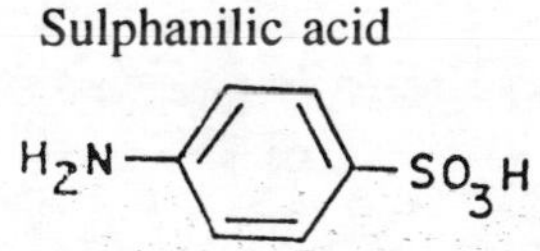

Thioureas

85.	Thiourea $H_2N\ CS\ NH_2$	Solid	m.p. 180°	Xanthyl, 136° Thiourea hydrochloride, 136°
86.	Phenylthiourea $C_6H_5\ NH—CS—NH_2$	Solid	m.p. 154°	Thiocarbanilide, 153°

Mercaptans

87.	Thiophenol C_6H_5SH	Liquid	b.p. 169°	Benzoate, 149° 2, 4-Dinitrophenyl sulphone, 149°

7. Preparation of Derivatives and Determination of their melting points:

After concluding the organic compound, the derivative is prepared (see chapter 11). The preparation of derivatives depend on the presence of the functional group. The determination of melting point of the derivative confirms the identity of the unknown organic compound.

11

Preparation of Derivatives

1. Carboxylic Acids

(a) Amide : Shake the acid (0.5 g) with phosphorous pentachloride (1.5 ml) or thionyl chloride (1.5 ml) till the vigorous reaction ceases. Warm the solution gently and then cool it. Now add cautiously concentrated ammonia solution (10.0 ml), and when the vigorous reaction ceases, stir, cool and filter the product (acid amide). Wash the acid amide with cold water, crystallize from water and dry.

$$RCOOH + PCl_5 \longrightarrow RCOCl + POCl_3 + HCl$$

$$RCOCl + NH_4OH \longrightarrow RCONH_2 + HCl + H_2O$$

(b) p–Nitrobenzyl Ester : Dissolve a small amount of the compound in minimum amount of water or alcohol. Add a drop of phenolphthalein followed by 20% aqueous potassium solution till a permanent red colour is obtained. Now add a little amount of the carboxylic acid till red colour disappears and then evaporate the contents to dryness. Add p-nitrobenzyl chloride (0.5 g), water (2 ml) and alcohol (6 ml) to the solid mass. Reflux the contents for half an hour, cool and add water (5 ml). Filter the product, wash with cold water and crystallize from alcohol.

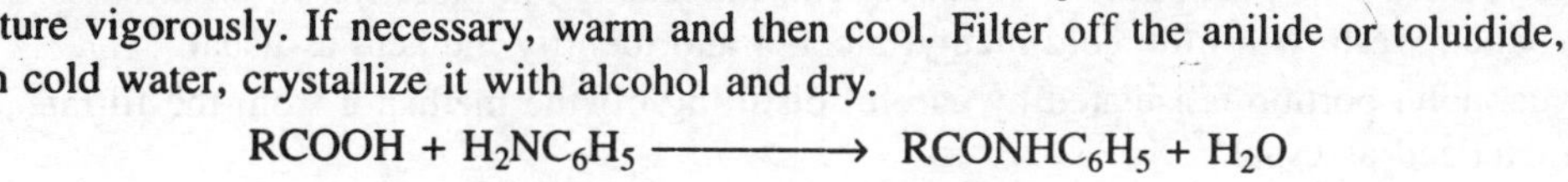

p—Nitrobenzyl chloride p—Nitrobenzyl ester

(c) Anilide or p-Toluidide : Shake the solution of an acid (0.5 g) with phosphorus pentachloride (0.5 ml) or thionyl chloride (1.5 ml) till the vigorous reaction ceases. Warm the solution gently and cool it. Add nearly one ml of aniline or p—toluidine and shake the reaction mixture vigorously. If necessary, warm and then cool. Filter off the anilide or toluidide, wash it with cold water, crystallize it with alcohol and dry.

$$RCOOH + \underset{\text{Aniline}}{H_2NC_6H_5} \longrightarrow \underset{\text{Anilide}}{RCONHC_6H_5} + H_2O$$

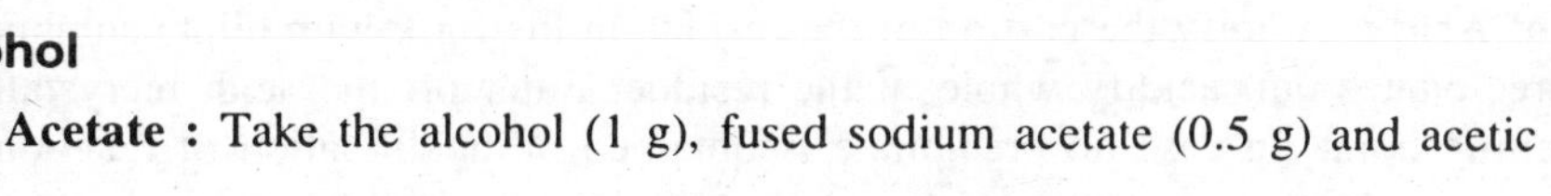

p—Toluidine p—Toluidide

2. Alcohol

(a) Acetate : Take the alcohol (1 g), fused sodium acetate (0.5 g) and acetic anhydride (5

ml) in a conical flask. Shake and heat the mixture on a water bath for 30 minutes. Transfer the warm solution into ice cold water (75 ml) with vigorous shaking. Keep the solution for sometime and filter the product. Wash with water and crystallize from alcohol.

$$ROH + (CH_3CO)_2O \xrightarrow{CH_3COONa} ROCOCH_3 + CH_3COOH$$

(b) Benzoate : Take the alcohol (1 ml), acetone (10 ml), benzoyl chloride (5 ml) and aqueous sodium hydroxide solution (50 ml) in a small flask. Cool, cork and shake the flask vigorously till the odour of benzoyl chloride disappears. Filter off the solid compound, wash well with water and crystallize from alcohol.

$$ROH + ClCOC_6H_5 \longrightarrow ROCOC_6H_5 + HCl$$

(c) 3, 5-Dinitrobenzoate : Dissolve the dry alcohol (0.5 g) in dry pyridine (5 ml). Add to this, solution of 3. 5-dinitrobenzoyl chloride. Reflux the mixture for about 30 minutes, cool and pour into dilute hydrochloric acid (30 ml) when 3, 5-dinitrobenzoate separates out. Wash the solid product with dilute sodium bicarbonate solution and then recrystallize from ethanol, aqueous ethanol or benzene.

ROH +

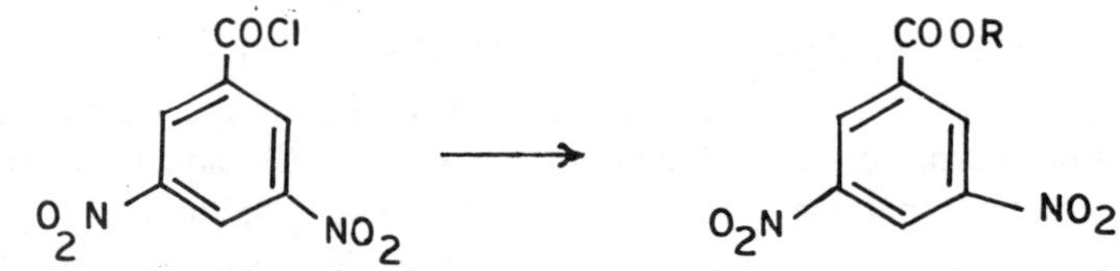

\+ HCl

Alcohol   3, 5-Dinitrobenzoyl Chloride   3, 5-Dinitrobenzoate

3. Esters

The most general derivatives of esters are their hydrolyzed products, acids and alcohols or phenols.

(a) Hydrolysis by Sodium Methoxide : Dissolve sodium (1 g) in pure methyl alcohol (10 ml) by warming in a dry flask fitted with a reflux condenser. Cool the solution and then treat it with the ester (1 g) and water (0.5 ml). A precipitate of carboxylic acid often separates out immediately; in case no precipitate is obtained, boil the reaction mixture for 30-60 minutes. Filter off the product, wash with little cold methyl alcohol and identify the acid as usual.

The alcoholic portion is isolated by careful distilling off the methanol from the filtrate. It is then characterized as usual.

(b) Hydrolysis by Aqueous Alkali : Take the ester (5 gm) in 30% potassium hydroxide solution (40 ml) in a conical flask. Boil the contents under reflux until hydrolysis is completed as indicated by a change in odour or appearance of mixture.

Isolation of Alcohol : Distill off a test portion of the liquid, separate the distillate with potassium carbonate, in case a distinct layer of alcohol separates out on standing; remove this layer, dry it with anhydrous potassium carbonate and identify the alcohol.

Isolation of Acid : Acidify the portion of the residue in the flask with dilute sulphuric acid, in case acid precipitates out, acidify whole of the residue. Filter off the acid, recrystallize and identify by melting point. In case no precipitate is obtained on acidification of reaction liquor, neutralize it to phenolphtholein and use the alkali salt of the acid for preparing a suitable derivative.

4. Aldehydes and Ketones

(a) Oxime :

(i) For Aldehydes and Aliphatic Ketones : Dissolve hydroxylamine hydrochloride (0.5 g) and hydrated sodium acetate (0.5 g) in water (3 ml). Add to it carbonyl compound (0.5 g), heat the mixture on the water bath and add ethanol dropwise with shaking until a clear solution is obtained. Continue refluxing to complete the reaction. Cool the product when the derivative will crystallize out.

(ii) For Aromatic and Some Cyclic Ketones : Dissolve the ketone (1 g) and hydroxylamine hydrochloride (0.6 g) in a mixture of ethanol (3 ml) and water (1 ml). Add sodium hydroxide (1 g), shake the mixture, and reflux for 30 minutes. Cool the reaction mixture, add water (20 ml) and shake. Filter the unchanged ketone, if any, and acidify the filtrate with dilute hydrochloric acid. Filter off the oxime.

(b) Semicarbozone

Dissolve semicarbazide hydrochloride (0.5 g) and hydrated sodium acetate (0.75 g) in water (5 ml). To the resulting solution, add the carbonyl compound (0.5 g) and shake well. In case a clear solution is not obtained, methanol is added dropwise, with shaking. The mixture is shaken and allowed to stand when the precipitate of semicarbazene will separate out, if not, heat the solution on water bath for 10 minutes and cool. Filter off the semicarbazone and recrystallize it from ethanol, glacial acetic acid or benzene.

$$\underset{}{>C=O} + \underset{\text{Semicarbazide}}{H_2NCONHNH_2} \longrightarrow \underset{\text{semicarbazone}}{>C=N\text{–}CONHNH_2}$$

5. Carbohydrates

(a) Osazone : Take the powdered sugar (0.5 g) in a clean tube. In another test tube, dissolve phenylhydrazine hydrochloride (0.4 g) and crystalline sodium acetate (0.6 g) in cold water (4 ml) and add this solution to sugar. Loosely cork the test tube, immerse it in a boiling water bath with periodical shaking, and note the exact time required for the first appearance of a turbidity or precipitate of osazone. Cool the solution, filter the precipitate and recrystallize it from 50% alcohol.

(b) Acetate : Dissolve the carbohydrate (0.5 g), powdered anhydrous sodium acetate (0.5 g) and acetic anhydride (3 ml) in glacial acetic acid (5 ml) by refluxing on a water bath. Further heat the solution for 2 hours. Pour cautiously the hot reaction mixture in cold water (25 ml) and stir the solution vigorously to decompose the excess of acetic anhydride. Filter off the product, wash with cold water and recrystallize from alcohol.

(c) Oxime : See carbonyl compounds.

$$\begin{array}{c} CHO \\ | \\ CHOH \\ | \\ R \end{array} \quad \text{or} \quad \begin{array}{c} CH_2OH \\ | \\ CO \\ | \\ R \end{array} \quad \xrightarrow{H_2NOH} \quad \begin{array}{c} CH=NOH \\ | \\ CHOH \\ | \\ R \end{array} \quad \text{or} \quad \begin{array}{c} CH_2OH \\ | \\ C{=}NOH \\ | \\ R \end{array}$$

6. Phenols

(a) Acetate : Since the acetate of monohydric phenols are usually liquids, acetates are prepared only in the case of polyhydric phenols and in naphthols.

Take the phenolic compound (1 g) in a clean dry test tube, add acetic anhydride (2.5 ml) and a drop of concentrated sulphuric acids.. Cork the tube, shake it vigorously for 4-5 minute and then transfer the reaction mixture to cold water (5 ml). Stir the contents with a glass rod till the oil solidifies..Filter, wash with water and recrystallize from hot water or dilute alcohol.

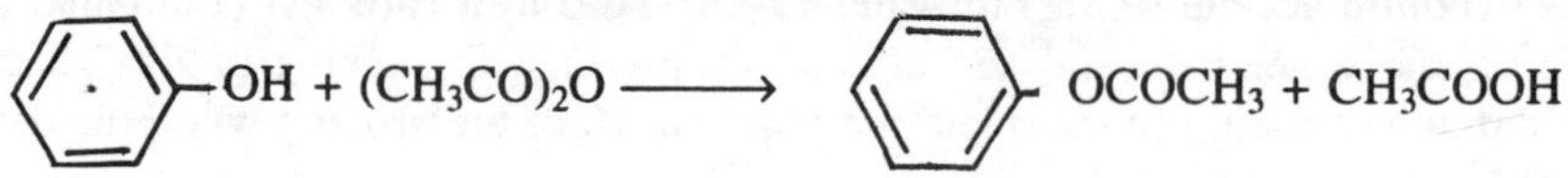

Phenol Acetate

(b) Benzoate : Dissolve the phenol (1.0 g) in acetone (5 ml) and add benzoyl chloride (2.5 ml). Add aqueous sodium hydroxide (10 ml) gradually with cooling and shaking, then further add NaOH solution (40 ml). Stopper the tube or the flask and shake vigorously till the odour of benzoyl chloride has disappeared. The final solution should be alkaline to litmus. Filter the solid benzoyl derivative, wash first with dilute hydrochloric acid, then with cold water, and recrystallize from alcohol, acetone (in case of resorcinol and p–naphthol) or benzene (in case of quinol and phloroglucinol).

$$\underset{\text{Phenol}}{Ar{-}OH} + \underset{\text{Benzoyl chloride}}{ClCOC_6H_5} \longrightarrow \underset{\text{Benzoate}}{ArOCOC_6H_5} + HCl$$

(c) Bromo Derivative: Dissolve or suspend the phenol (200 g) in water (100 ml) and then add a solution of bromine (20 ml) in glacial acetic acid (10 ml) dropwise with vigorous shaking until faint yellow colour persists. Filter off the precipitated bromo derivative, wash thoroughly with water and recrystallize with dilute alcohol.

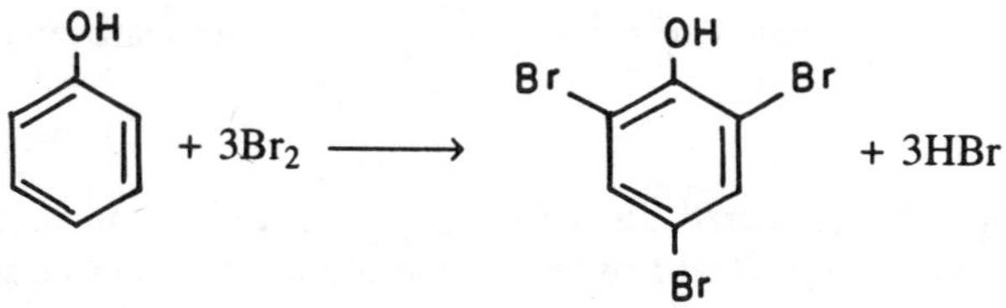

Phenol Tribromophenol

7. Primary And Secondary Amines

(a) Acetyl derivative :

(i) For Primary Amines : Suspend the amine (0.5 g) in water (0.5 ml), add glacial acetic acid (0.5 ml) and acetic anhydride (1.5 ml) dropwise with shaking. If the mixture does not dissolve warm spontaneously, it is heated cautiously over a small flame for 15 minute. Cool the reaction mixture. If the oil does not solidify, stir with glass rod and cool in an ice bath. Filter off the acetyl derivative and recrystallize from water or aqueous ethyl alcohol.

$$R{-}NH_2 \xrightarrow[CH_3COOH]{(CH_3CO)_2O} R{-}NHCOCH_3$$

(ii) For Secondary Amine : Warm a mixture of the amine (0.5 g) and acetic anhydride (0.5g) on the water bath for 5-10 minutes. Cool, add water (3 ml) and stir the mixture until the derivative is solidified.

$$R_2{-}NH + (CH_3CO)_2O \xrightarrow{\text{Heat}} R_2{-}NCOCH_3 + CH_3COOH$$

(b) Benzoyl Derivative :

Suspend the compound (0.5 g) in 5% sodium hydroxide solution (10 ml) in a small conical flask. Add dropwise benzoyl chloride (1 ml), the flask should be well stoppered and shaken vigorously with addition of reagents. The reaction mixture should be kept cool throughout the addition. Finally, shake the reaction mixture vigorously for 5-10 minute and filter off the product. Wash the derivative with water and recrystallize from alcohol.

$$R—NH_2 + C_6H_5COCl \longrightarrow R—NHCOC_6H_5 + HCl$$

$$R_2—NH + C_6H_5COCl \longrightarrow R_2—N\ COC_6H_5 + HCl$$

(c) 2, 4-Dinitrophenyl Derivative :

Take the amine (1 g), 2, 4-dinitro- chlorobenzene (1 g), ethanol (10 ml) and a slight excess of anhydrous potassium carbonate or anhydrous sodium acetate in a conical flask. Reflux the contents after thorough mixing for 30 minutes. Pour the contents into cold water and filter off the product. Wash the derivative with water and recrystallize from alcohol.

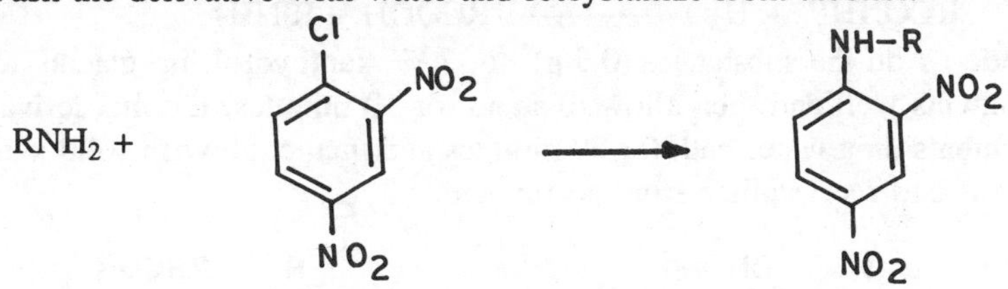

Amine 2, 4-Dinitro chlorobenzene 2, 4-Dinitro phenyl derivative

(d) Bromo Derivative :

Few aromatic amines give easily identifiable product on bromination (see phenols).

(e) Picrate : See Phenols

$$R—NH_2 + C_6H_2(NO_2)_3\ OH \longrightarrow R—NH_2.C_6H_2(NO_2)_3.OH$$

Picric acid Picrate

8. Tertiary Amines

(a) Methiodide : Take the tertiary amine (0.5 g) in a test tube and treat it with methyl iodide (0.5 ml) at room temperature. Keep the reaction mixture undisturbed for 5 minutes, then heat under reflex on the water bath for 5 minutes and finally cool in ice water. The quaternary salt will be crystallized out and, if not, scratch the sides of the tube with a glass rod. Recrystallization may be done from absolute alcohol, acetone or glacial acetic acid.

$$\rangle N— + CH_3I \longrightarrow \rangle N^+CH_3I^-$$

Tertiary Amine Methiodide

(b) Picrate : See Phenols

$$\rangle N— + C_6H_2(NO_2)_3OH \longrightarrow \rangle N.C_6H_2(NO_2)_3.OH$$

Picric acid picrate

(c) p-Nitroso Compound : Dissolve the amine (0.1 g) in an excess of 5 N hydrochloric acid (3 ml) and cool to 0° in an ice bath. Add cold sodium nitrite solution dropwise until only a very slight excess of nitroso acid is present. Filter off the crystalline product.

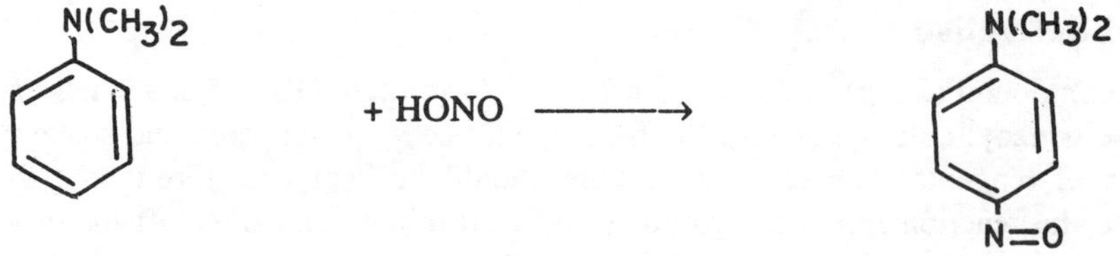

Dimethylaniline p-Nitrosodimethylaniline

9. Amides, Imides And Anilides

(a) Hydrolysis : Take the compound (0.5 g) and excess of 25 % sodium hydroxide solution in a conical flask fitted with a reflux condenser. Reflux the contents until all ammonia has been driven off and then cool. Add concentrated hydrochloric acid dropwise till the reaction mixture is strongly acidic and then acid separates out as a derivative. Filter and recrystallize from alcohol.

$$RONH_2 + H_2O \longrightarrow RCOOH + NH_3$$

$$RCONHR' + H_2O \longrightarrow RCOOH + R'NH_2$$

(b) Xanthylamide : Add the substance (0.5 g) to 7 % xanthydrol in glacial acetic acid (7 ml). Shake the contents well and then allow to stand for 10 minutes. If solid derivative is not obtained, heat the contents on a water bath for 30 minutes and then cool when solid xanthylamide is obtained. Filter it off and recrystallize from acetic acid.

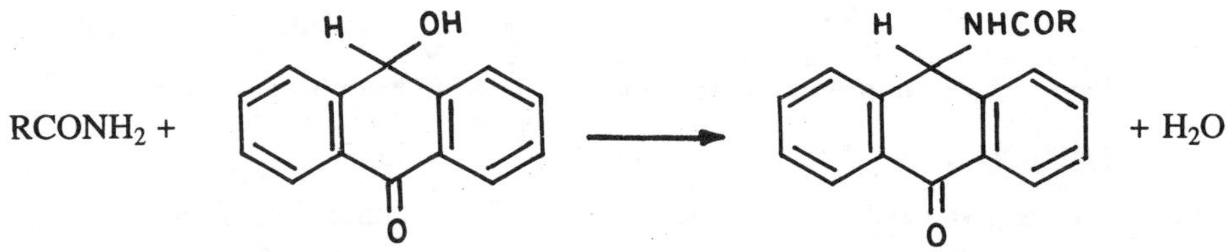

Xanthydrol Xanthylamide

10. Sulphonic Acids

(a) Sulphonamide : Mix dry sulphonic acid (1 g) and with phosphorus pentachloride (2 g). Heat the mixture on a oil bath at 150°C for about 30 minutes. When the reaction is completed, cool the contents and treat with cold water (15 ml). Stir and wash the sulphonyl chloride twice with cold water by decantation. Now add concentrated ammonia solution (5 ml) with stirring. Heat the reaction mixture on a water bath for 5-10 minutes and then cool. The amide will start crystallizing out. Recrystallize the derivative from water or aqueous alcohol.

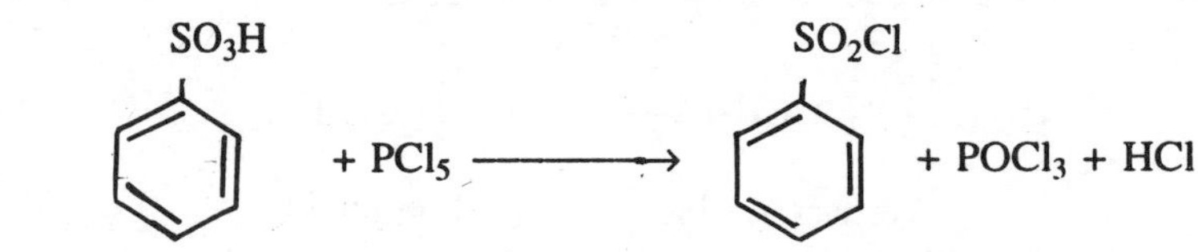

Sulphonic acid Sulphonyl chloride

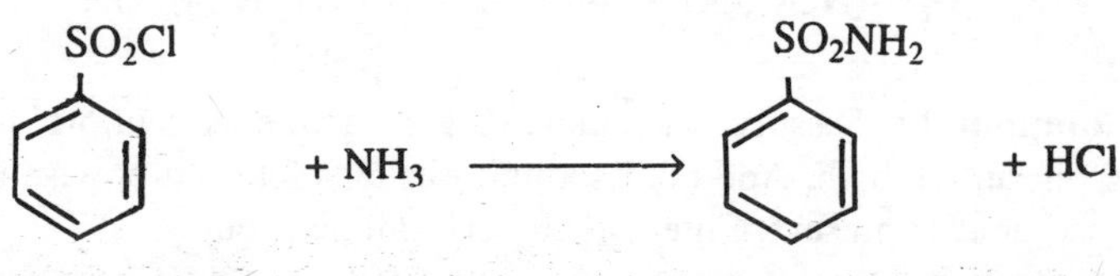

Sulphonyl chloride Benzenesulphonamide

(b) Sulphonanilide : Prepare the sulphonyl chloride as above in method (a). Dissolve it in acetone and treat with pure aniline (0.5 ml) dissolved in acetone together with dilute sodium hydroxide solution (25 ml). Shake the mixture for 10 minutes and extract with ether to remove excess of aniline. Acidify the product, filter and recrystallize from dilute alcohol.

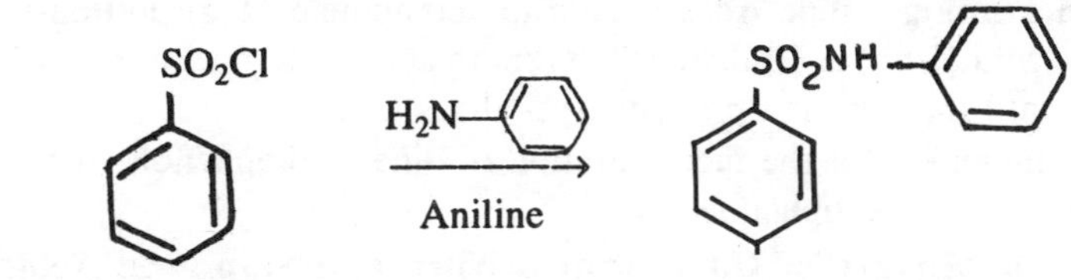

Benzene sulphonyl chloride — Sulphananilide

11. Hydrocarbons

(a) Nitration of Halogen Hydrocarbons : Take the compound (1 g or 1 ml) in a dry test tube, add to it concentrated nitric acid (1.5 ml) and concentrated sulphuric acid (1.5 ml). Place the test tube in boiling water for 5 minute with occasional shaking. Cool, add water (1 ml) and shake. Filter off the product, wash with cold water and crystallize from alcohol.

(b) Picrate : See phenols

$$C_{10}H_8 + C_6H_2(NO_2)_3OH \longrightarrow C_{10}H_8C_6H_2(NO_2)_8\,OH$$

Naphthalene Picric acid Naphthalene picrate

(c) Oxidation products : (By $KMnO_4$) : Add xylene (1.5 g) or ethyl benzene (1.5 g) or toluene (0.75 g) or a substituted toluene (0.75 g)) of the compound to a solution of sodium carbonate (1 g) and potassium permanganate (3 g) in water (50 ml). Reflux the mixture until potassium permanganate colour disappears. Filter off precipitated manganese dioxide and acidify the filtrate with concentrated hydrochloric acid. Filter off and identify the precipitated acid.

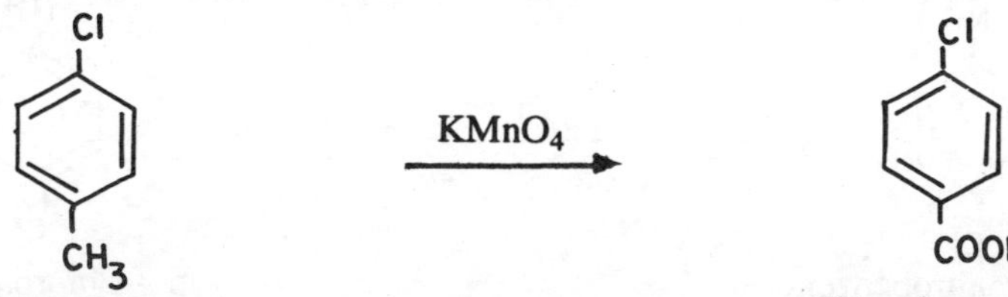

p-Chlorotoluene — p-Chlorobenzoic acid

12. Nitro Compounds

Aromatic hydrocarbons and most of their halogeno and nitroderivatives can be nitrated with the help of suitable nitrating mixture. Infact there is no general method for the preparation of nitroderivatives since the experimental conditions vary with the compound to be nitrated.

(a) Nitro Derivative

(i) Nitration with Concentrated Nitric Acid : Add the compound (1 g) portion-wise with shaking to concentrated nitric acid (5 ml) at room temperature. Stir the mixture for 10 minutes and add some crushed ice when the product will be crystallized out either on standing or on scratching the sides of the test tube with a glass rod. Filter off the product, wash water and recrystallize.

[The above method is recommended for the mononitration of naphthalenes, alkylnaphthalenes, halogenonapthalenes and p—halogenophenols. For the mononitration of dihalogenobenzene and the dinitration of diphenyl, the mixture on adding the contents is warmed on a boiling water bath for 10 minutes, cooled and then worked as above].

(ii) Nitration with Fuming Nitric Acid : Add the compound (1 g) portion-wise and with shaking to fuming nitric acid (5 ml) at O°C. Stir the mixture at room temperature for 5-10 minutes, pour on to ice and stir until the nitration product crystallizes out.

The method is recommended for the mononitration of dihalogenophenols, for the dinitration of mesitylene, dibenzyl and halogenophenols.

(iii) Nitration with a Mixture of Concentrated Nitro and Sulphuric Acids : Add the compound (1 g) dropwise and with constant shaking to a mixture of concentrated sulphuric and nitric acids. Cool the solution either under tap or in ice cold water bath to 20—25°C. After standing for 10 minutes, pour the solution mixture on to ice and stir until the product solidifies.

The method is suitable for the dinitration of tetralin and anisole; for the mononitration of monohalogenobenzenes and for the dinitration of toluene, nitrophenols and o- and p-nitrotoluene and for the trinitration of dinitrophenols and o-nitroanisole.

(iv) Nitration with a Mixture of Fuming Nitric and Sulphuric Acids : Add the compound (1 g) dropwise to a mixture of fuming nitric acid (6 ml) and concentrated sulphuric acid (10 ml), with shaking. Heat the reaction mixture on a boiling water bath for 2-3 minutes, Cool, pour into ice-water and stir until the product solidifies.

The method is suitable for the nitration of nitrobenzene, for the dinitration of benzene, mono— and di-halogenobenzenes and of o- and p-nitrotoluenes, for the trinitration of m-xylene and for tetranitration of diphenylmethane.

(b) Amino Derivative

Nitro compounds can be easily reduced to the corresponding amino compounds in the presence of tin (or zinc) and hydrochloric acid, e.g.

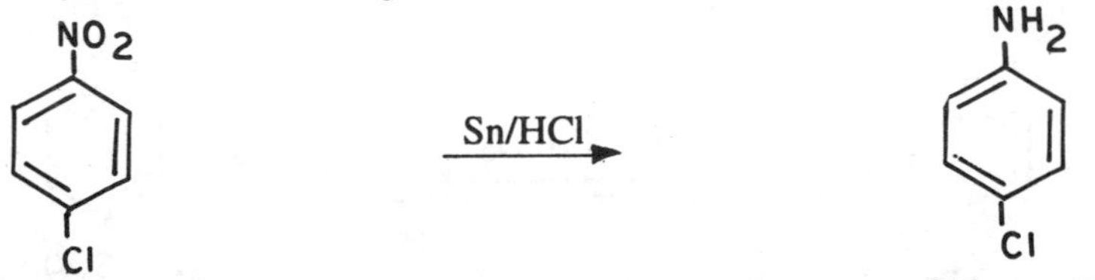

p—Chloronitrobenzene p—Chloroaniline

The corresponding amino derivative gives the derivatives of the amino group.

Place a small amount of the compound dissolved in alcohol in a conical flask. To this add tin pieces (2 g) and dilute hydrochloric acid (15-20 ml) in small instalments with constant shaking after each addition. Reflux the mixture on a boiling water bath for 10-15 minutes. Decent off the hot solution, dissolve the tin hydroxide with the help of dilute (40 %) sodium hydroxide solution and then extract the resulting solution several times with ether. Distil off the solvent ether and recrystallize the amino derivative with alcohol.

Derivatives of Thiols

Alkyl (or Aryl) 2, 4-Dinitrophenyl Sulphides (or Thioethers) : Dissolve the mercaptan (0.5 g) in rectified spirit (0-15 ml) and add 10 % sodium hydroxide solutions (2 ml). Mix the resulting sodium mercaptide solution with a solution of 2, 4-dinitrochlorobenzene (1 g) in of rectified spirit (5 ml). Reaction may occur immediately with precipitation of the thioether. In any case reflux the mixture for 10 minutes on a water bath in order to ensure the completeness of the reaction. Filter the hot solution rapidly; allow the solution to cool when the sulphide will crystallize out. Recrystallize from alcohol.

Derivatives of Thiourea

S–Benzylisothiouronium Chloride : Place a mixture of benzyl chloride (2 g), thiourea (1 g) and rectified spirit (3 ml) in a 50 ml round bottomed flask fitted with a reflux condenser. Warm on a water bath. A sudden exothermic reaction soon occurs and all the thiourea passes into solution. Reflux the resulting yellow solution for 30 minutes and then cool in ice. Filter off the white crystals and dry in the air. Concentrate the filtrate to half it original volume and thus obtain a further small crop of crystals. Recrystallize from 0.2 N hydrochloric acid.

$$\underset{\text{Thiourea}}{NH_2CSNH_2} + C_6H_5CH_2Cl \longrightarrow \underset{\text{δ-Benzyl isothiouronium chloride}}{\{C_6H_5CH_2—S—\underset{\underset{NH_2}{\|}}{C}—NH_2\}^+ \; Cl^-}$$

12

Identification Tests of Organic Drugs

The organic drugs are either obtained from natural sources or synthesized in laboratory. These drugs are identified on the bases of physical constants and chemical tests. Physical tests include determination of physical characters, e.g. shape, colour, solubility behaviour, specific rotation and boiling or melting point. Chemical tests are carried out to perform some colour reactions which are based on functional groups present in the molecule.

In the chapter identification tests are presented for some naturally occurring and synthetic organic drugs .

ASCORBIC ACID OR VITAMIN C

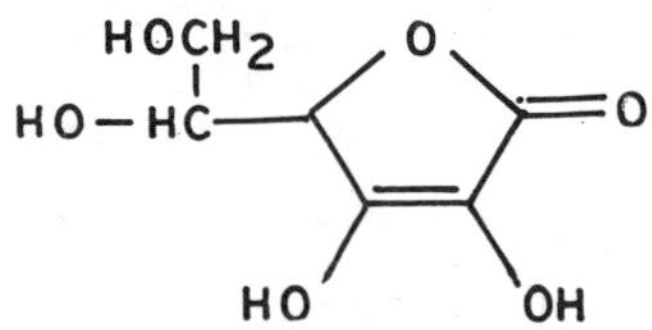

Ascorbic acid

Physical Properties

It is available as odourless, colourless crystals or white to pale yellow crystalline powder with acidic sour taste. It is freely soluble in water, slightly soluble in alcohol but insoluble in chloroform and ether.

Chemical Tests

1. Add 2% w/v solution of ascorbic acid (2 ml) to a few ml of 2, 6-dichloro-phenolindophenol solution, the solution is decolourized.
2. Dilute 2% w/v solution of ascorbic acid (1 ml) with water (5 ml), add one drop of freshly prepared sodium nitroprusside and dilute sodium hydroxide solution (2 ml). Add hydrochloric acid (0.6 ml) dropwise with shaking. The yellow colour turns blue.
3. Dilute 2% w/v solution of ascorbic acid (2 ml) with water (2 ml), add sodium bicarbonate (100 mg) and ferrous sulphate (20 mg), shake well. A deep violet colour is produced which disappears on adding dilute sulphuric acid (5 ml).

ASPIRIN
(Syn : Acetylsalicylic acid)

Chemical structure

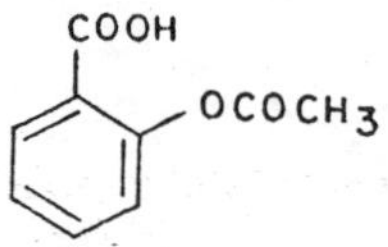

Aspirin

Physical Properties

It is an odourless, colourless or white crystalline powder with slightly acidic taste. It is slightly soluble in water but soluble in alcohol, chloroform and ether.

Chemical Tests

(i) Boil aspirin (0.5 g) with sodium hydroxide solution (10 ml) for 5 minutes, cool and acidify with dilute sulphuric acid (10 ml). White precipitate is produced and the odour of acetic acid is perceptible. Filter the precipitate, dissolve in water and add ferric chloride solution; a deep violet colour is produced.

This test is based on the hydrolysis of aspirin into salicylic acid and acetic acid. Salicylic acid gives deep violet colour with ferric chloride solution due to the presence of phenolic group.

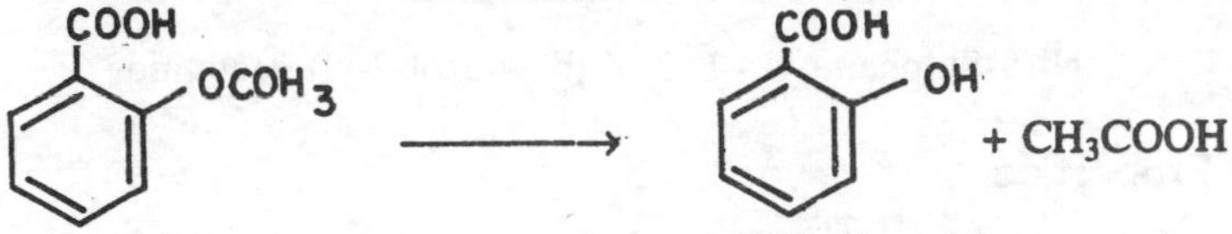

Aspirin Salicylic acid

(ii) Boil aspirin (0.5 g) with sodium hydroxide solution (10 ml) for 3 minutes, cool and acidify with dilute sulphuric acid (10 ml). A white precipitate is produced and the odour of acetic acid is perceptible. Filter, add alcohol (3 ml) and sulphuric to the filtrate and warm. The odour of ethyl acetate is perceptible.

Aspirin is hydrolyzed into insoluble salicylic acid and soluble acetic acid. On filtration, acetic acid appears in the filtrate which forms ester (ethyl acetate) by heating with alcohol in the presence of sulphuric acid

$$\underset{\text{Acetic acid}}{CH_3COOH} + \underset{\text{Ethanol}}{C_2H_5OH} \xrightarrow{H_2SO_4} \underset{\text{Ethyl acetate}}{CH_3COOC_2H_5}$$

Category: Analgesic, antipyretic and anti-inflammatory.

ANALGIN

Chemical structure.

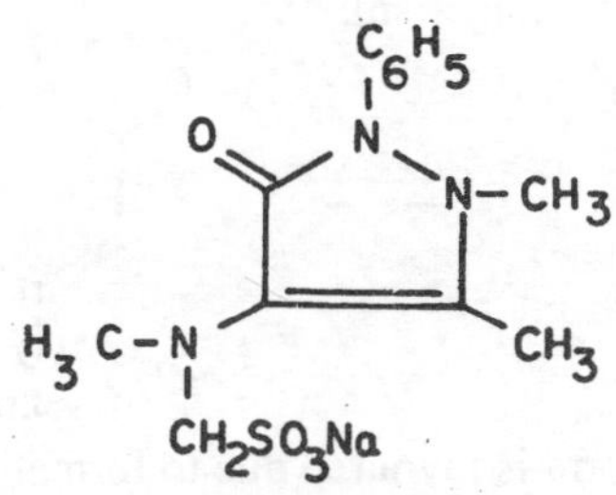

Analgin

Physical Properties

It is a white crystalline powder with a scarcely perceptible yellowish tinge, odourless, bitter taste. Is is soluble in water but insoluble in chloroform and solvent ether.

Chemical Test

(i) Add a few drops of water to analgin powder (100 mg), then add alcohol (5 ml) and dilute hydrochloric acid (0.5 ml). To this solution, add potassium iodate solution (5 ml); crimson colour is produced which deepens on further addition of potassium iodate solution.

(ii) Boil analgin (200 mg) with dilute hydrochloric acid (2 ml), the characteristic odour of sulphur dioxide is produced followed by formaldehyde.

Category : Analgesic

ACETAZOLAMIDE

Chemical structure :

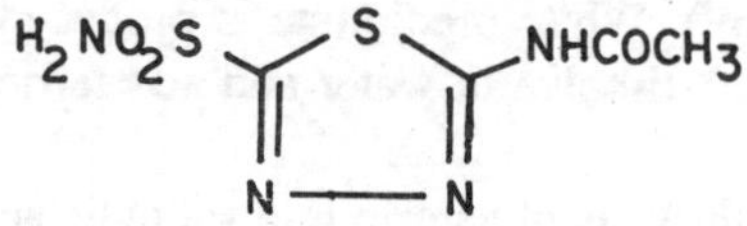

Acetazolamide

N-(5-Sulphamoyl –1, 3, 4-thiadiazol-2-yl) acetamide

Physical Properties

It is white or yellowish white, odourless, tasteless crystalline powder. It is slightly soluble in water and alcohol but insoluble in chloroform and solvent ether.

Chemical Tests

(i) Triturate acetazolamide (500 mg) with water (5 ml), add sodium hydroxide solution (1 ml) to make alkaline, zinc powder (200 mg), hydrochloric acid (0.5 ml) and mix well. Hydrogen sulphide gas is evolved which is recognized by its characteristic odour.

(ii) To acetazolamide (25 mg), add water (5 ml), sodium hydroxide (4 ml) and copper sulphate (2 ml). A bluish green colour or precipitate is produced.

Category : diuretic, antiepileptic

BARBITURATES

Barbiturates are cyclic ureides, used as hypnotic and sedative. They are found in two isomeric enolic and ketonic forms due to tautomerism.

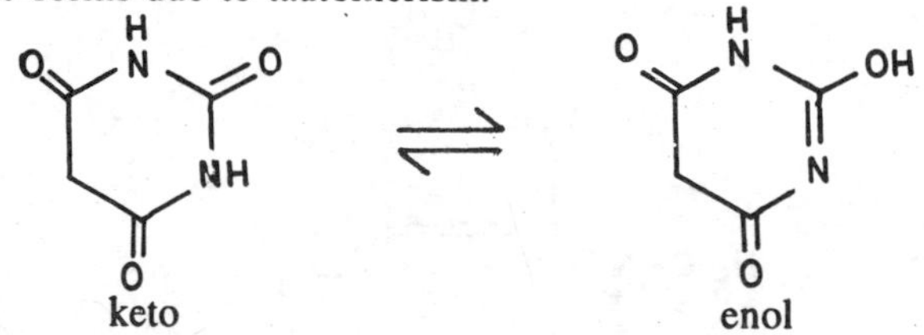

keto enol

In alkaline solution, enolic form is favoured due to formation of salt. Substitution in barbituric acid at position 5 by alkyl or aryl group gives the various type of barbiturates, differing in onset and duration of action.

Physical Properties

Barbiturates are odourless, colourless or white crystalline powders with acidic character. They are slightly soluble in water but their corresponding sodium salt are soluble in water.

Free barbiturates are identified by melting point. For the sodium salt (which decomposes without any definite melting point), add hydrochloric acid, filter the precipitate, warm with water, dry and take melting point.

Chemical Test

(i) Boil a barbiturate (200 mg) with sodium hydroxide solution (10 ml); ammonia is evolved.
(ii) Dissolve a barbiturate (180 mg) in a mixture of sodium hydroxide (0.5 ml) and 10% w/v solution of pyridine (2 ml); add further pyridine solution (8 ml), copper sulphate solution (1 ml) with pyridine and set aside for 10 minutes, a specific colour is produced depending on barbiturate. For sodium salt, it is not necessary to add sodium hydroxide solution.

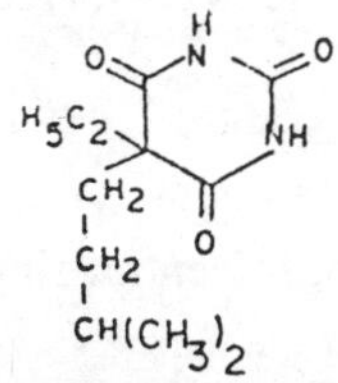

Amylobarbitone
Reddish violet

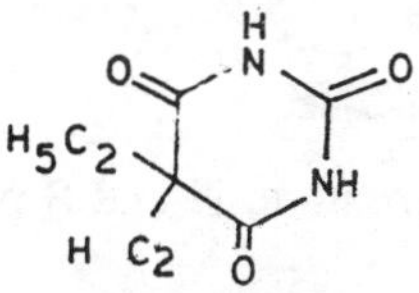

Barbitone
(lilac)

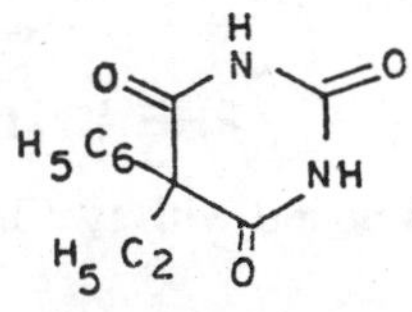

Phenobarbitone
(lilac)

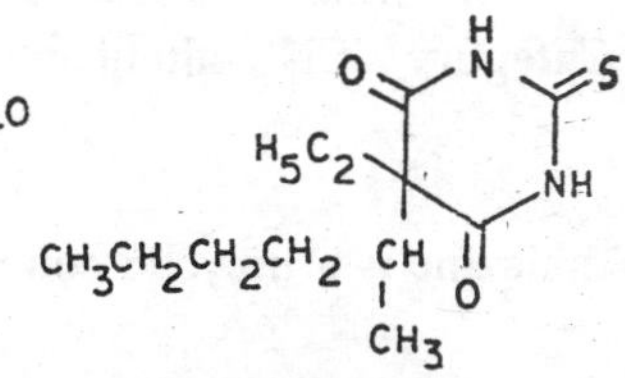

Thiopentone
(Green)

(iii) Barbiturates may be identified by preparation of their derivatives. For example, official identification test of amylobarbitone is based on preparation of its nitrobenzyl derivative by reaction with p-nitrobenzyl chloride.

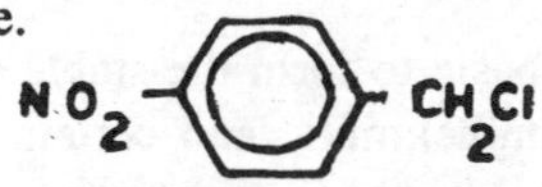

p-Nitrobenzyl chloride

Triturate amylobarbitone (600 mg) with anhydrous sodium carbonate (150 mg) and water (5 ml). Add a solution of p-nitrobenzyl chloride (450 mg) in 10 ml of alcohol and warm on a water bath for 30 minutes. Cool, allow to stand for one hour, filter and wash the residue with sodium hydroxide (10 ml) and then water. The residue after recrystallization melts at about 150° or at about 168°.

Category : Hypnotic and sedative

CAFFEINE

Chemical structure

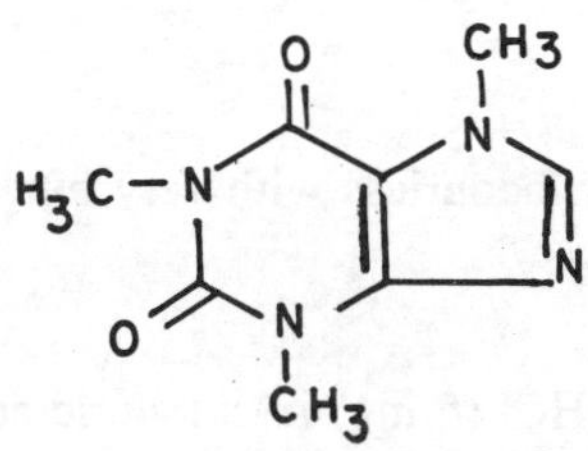

Caffeine (1, 3, 7-Trimethylxanthine)

Physical Properties

It occurs as silky white crystals or white glistening needles or white crystalline powder, odourless with bitter taste. It is slightly soluble in water and alcohol but freely soluble in chloroform and boiling water.

Chemical Tests

(i) Take caffeine (10 mg) in a porcelain dish, add hydrochloric acid (1 ml) and potassium chlorate (100 mg) and evaporate to dryness on a water bath. Expose the residue to the vapours of dilute ammonia solution; a purple colour is produced which disappears on addition of a solution of alkali.

(ii) To a saturated solution of caffeine, add a few drops of tannic acid solution; a white precipitate is produced which is soluble in excess of the reagent.

(iii) To a saturated solution of caffeine (5 ml), add 0.1 N iodine solution (1.5 ml) untill solution remains clear. Add a few drops of dilute hydrochloric acid; a brown precipitate is formed. Neutralize with sodium hydroxide solution, the precipitate is dissolved.

Category : CNS stimulant

PHENOTHIAZINE

Phenothiazine is a tricyclic compound with two heteroatom, N and S present in central ring.

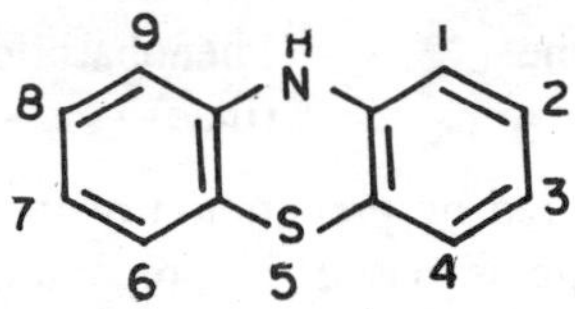

Phenothiazine is not sufficiently basic to form the stable salts with acid. Phenothiazine itself is used in veterinary practice as an anthelmintic and certain of its derivatives are of medicinal importance, e.g. chropromazine hydrochloride (antihistaminic drug).

Chloropromazine Hydrochloride

Chemical structure :

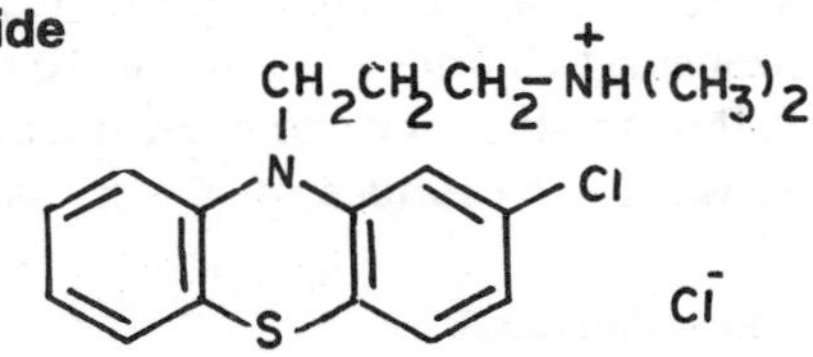

Chloropromazine hydrochloride

(3-(2-Chlorophenothiazin-10yl) propyl-N, N-dimethyl ammonium chloride)

Physical Properties

It is a white or creamy white powder, odourless with very bitter taste.

Chemical Test

(i) Dissolve chloropromazine HCl (5 mg) in sulphuric acid (5 ml). A cherry red colour is produced which darkens slowly on standing. A portion of this on warming changes through brown to magenta, the remaining portion on addition of 0.1 N potassium dichromate (0.2 ml) changes to brownish red.

(ii) Dissolve the drug (5 mg) in water (5 ml) and add one drop of ferric chloride solution; a stable red colour is produced.

Category : Central nervous system depressant, transquillizer and antiemetic

SULPHONAMIDES

Sulphanilamide, p-aminobenzene sulphonamide, is the simplest sulphonamide.

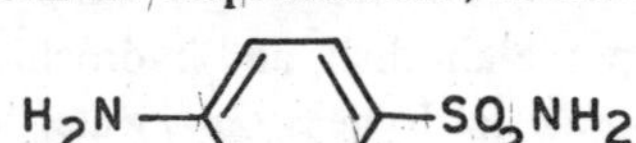

The derivatives of sulphanilamide, used in medicine, may have variable substituents in place of hydrogen of sulphonamido group, e.g. sulphadiazine contain pyrimidine moiety.

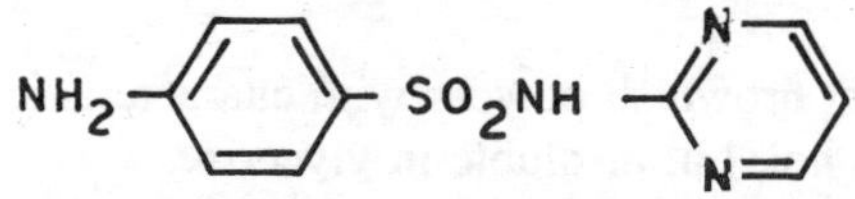

The p-amino group in essential for its activity and one of the hydrogen can be replaced only by such group which can provide again free amino group in the body. For example, phthalyl sulphathiazole and succinyl sulphathiazole.

Sulphonamides have the antibacterial activity.

Sulpha drugs containing free amino group can be identified by diazotization followed by coupling with alkaline β—naphthol solution to give dyes of orange-red colour.

Some sulphanilamide can be identified by the product of hydrolysis. For example, the sulphacetamide on heating with 95% alcoholic solution in the presence of sulphuric acid give the odour of ethyl acetate. Sulphaguanidine on alkaline hydrolysis forms ammonia.

Many sulphanilamide are characterized by the colours of copper complexes made by the action of copper sulphate in the alkaline solution.

SULPHACETAMIDE

Chemical structure

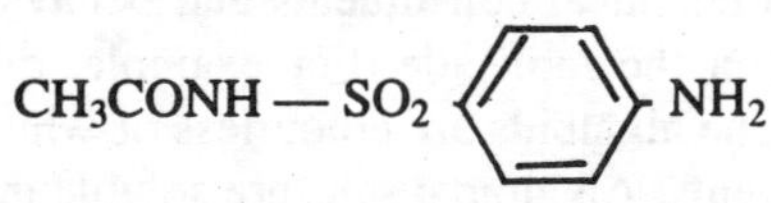

p—Acetylaminobenzene sulphonamide

Physical Properties

It is a white or yellowish white crystalline powder, odourless, with acidic and saline taste.

Chemical Test

(i) Dissolve sulphacetamide (50 mg) in warm dilute hydrochloric acid (2 ml) and pour the solution in β—naphthol (2 ml) containing sodium acetate (1 g). An orange precipitate is formed.

Sulphacetamide contains free amino group. Therefore, it is diazotized and coupled with β-naphthol to form an orange dye.

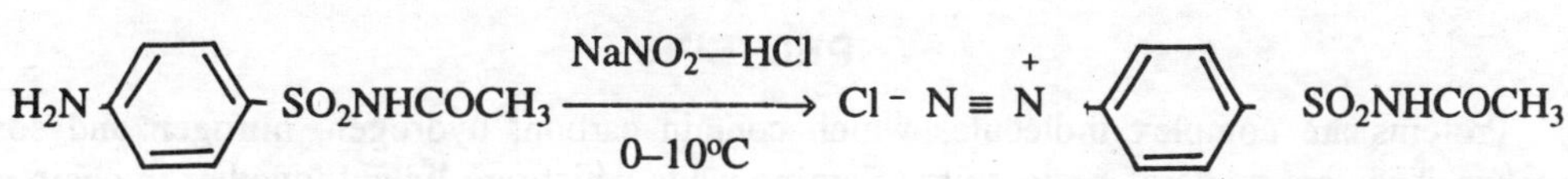

Sulphacetamide Diazotized sulphacetamide

(ii) Heat sulphacetamide with alcohol and sulphuric acid. Ethyl acetate, recognizable by its odour, is produced.

(iii) Place sulphacetamide (500 mg) in a test tube, heat gently until it melts and then boil. An oily liquid, which has characteristic odour of acetamide, condenses on the wall of the test tube.

Catetory : Antibacterial

TANNIC ACID

Tannic acid is obtained from the galls of various species of *Quercus* (Family : Fagaceae) or other vegetable sources.

Physical Properties

It is a yellowish white or light brownish powder with characteristic odour and astringent taste. It is soluble in water and alcohol, but insoluble in glycerin.

Chemical Test

(i) A solution of tannic acid gives precipitates with a solution of gelatin, albumin and certain alkaloids.

(ii) A solution of tannic acid gives a bluish-black colour with solution of ferric chloride. On addition of dilute sulphuric acid, the colour disappears and a yellowish brown precipitate is formed.

Category : Astringent.

ALKALOIDS

Alkaloids are basic nitrogenous compounds with definite physiological and pharmacological activity. They contain atleast one nitrogen in a ring except few exception like ephedrine.

They differ considerably in chemical constituents and behaviour. They are classified on the basis of basic skeleton present in the molecule. For example, quinine contains quinoline ring; atropine contains tropane ring. The alkaloids are colourless or white crystalline mass, insoluble in water but soluble in organic solvents. Alkaloidal salts are soluble in water and insoluble in organic solvent.

They are identified on the basis of their melting point and generalized chemical tests which are as follows:

(i) Add few drops of Dragendorff's reagent to a solution of alkaloid (2 ml) or its salt; orange-red precipitate is produced.

(ii) Add few drops of Mayer's reagent to a solution of alkaloid; a white-yellowish precipitate is produced.

(iii) Add few drops of solution in potassium iodide to a solution of alkaloid, a brown precipitate is produced.

(iv) Add few drops of saturated solution of picric acid to a solution of alkaloid, a pale yellow precipitate is produced.

PROTEINS

Proteins are complex molecules which contain carbon, hydrogen, nitrogen and sometime sulphur. They are made of basic units of amino acids which are linked together in chain or rings through peptide bonds. Carboxylic group of one amino acid is joined with amino group of another amino acid.

$$\begin{array}{ccccc} R_1 - \underset{\displaystyle NH_2}{\underset{|}{CH}} - COOH & + & NH_2 - \underset{\displaystyle COOH}{\underset{|}{CH}} - R_2 & \longrightarrow & R_1 - \underset{\displaystyle NH_2}{\underset{|}{CH}} - CO\,NH - \underset{\displaystyle COOH}{\underset{|}{CH}} - R_2 \\ \text{Amino acid} & & \text{Amino acid} & & \text{Peptide} \end{array}$$

Proteins are amphoteric in nature. At some definite pH, characteristic of each protein, the positive and negative charges are exactly balanced and the molecules do not migrate in an electrical field. This condition is known as 'isoelectric point' and at this pH the protein has its least solubility.

Proteins are examined by the following colour reaction, e.g.

1. **Biuret Reaction :** To alkaline solution of protein (2 ml), a dilute solution of copper sulphate is added. A red or violet colour is formed with peptides containing at least two peptide linkages. A dipeptide does not respond this test.
2. **Xanthroproteic Reaction :** Proteins usually form a yellow colour on warming with concentrated nitric acid. This colour becomes orange when the solution is made alkaline. The colour is due to nitration of aromatic ring containing amino acids like phenylalamine and tyrosine.
3. **Ninhydrin Test :** To an aqueous solution of a protein, an alcoholic solution of ninhydrin is added and then heated. Red to violet colour is formed.

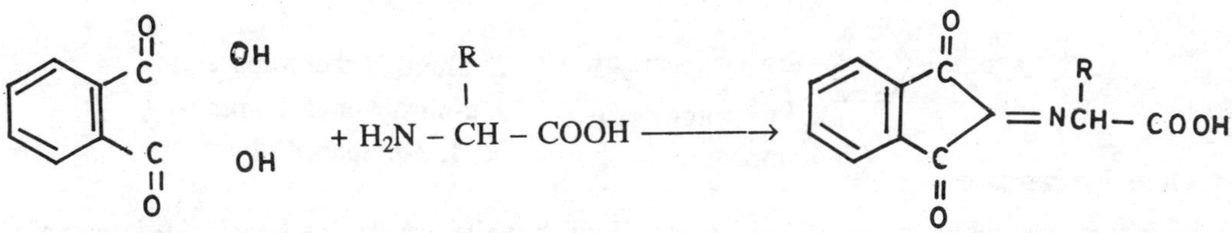

Ninhydrin — Amino acid — Coloured compound

4. **Nitroprusside Test :** Proteins containing sulphur atom form red colour with nitroprusside solution.
5. **Lead Sulphide Test :** Alkaline solution of sulphur containing protein, on addition of lead acetate, produces a black precipitate.

AMINO ACIDS

An amino acid is the hydrolytic product of protein. They are characterized by the presence of amino and carboxylic groups together. They are aliphatic or aromatic in nature. They are detected by following chemical test.

1. Amino acids give red to violet colour with ninhydrin.
2. Phenolic amino acids give red colour on addition of ferric chloride solution.
3. Aromatic amino acids undergo diazotization with nitrous acid which couple with alkaline β-naphthol solution to give red coloured aze dye.
4. **Sorensen Test** (only for aliphatic amino acid) : Take the compound (0.5 g) and dissolve in water or alcohol. Add two drops of phenolphthalein and then dilute sodium hydroxide solution till pink colour is obtained. In the other test tube take the similar things in a similar order only with the difference that the amino acid is replaced by 40% formalin solution. Add the solution from the second test tube to the first; the disappearance of the pink colour is the indication of amino acid.

GLYCINE

$$H_2N — CH_2 — COOH$$

Physical properties

Glycine is the simplest amino acid. It is a colourless solid. It is readily soluble in water.

Chemical Test

1. Glycine contain the basic group, —NH_2 as well as the acidic group —COOH, hence it

forms salt with both alkalies and acids.

2. Its aqueous solution gives red colour on addition of 2 or 3 drops of ninhydrin solution.
3. To the compound (2 ml), add 2 drops of phenolphthalein solution, 2 drops of dilute aqueous sodium hydroxide solution and 2—3 ml of neutralized alcohol (3 ml). The pink colour disappears.
4. Glycine reacts with nitrous acid like primary amines, the NH_2 group is displaced by hydroxyl group and glycollic acid is formed.

$$NH_2CH_2COOH + HNO_2 \rightarrow \underset{\text{Glycollic acid}}{HOCH_2COOH} + N_2 + H_2O$$

CHLORAMPHENICOL

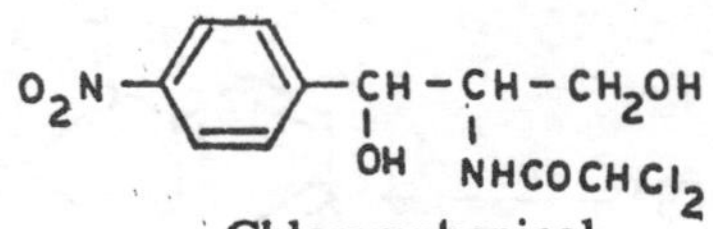

Chloramphenicol

D-Threo-N-dichloroacetyl 1-p-nitrophenyl-2-amino-1, 3-propanediol

Physical Properties

It occurs as a fine, white to greyish white or yellowish white, crystalline powder. It is odourless with bitter taste.

Chloramphenicol is slightly soluble in water; freely soluble in alcohol and in acetone; slightly soluble in solvent ether.

Chemical test

1. Ferric chloride test for nitro group : To the sample (10 mg), dissolved in 50% alcohol (1 ml) and 0.1 N calcium chloride solution (3 ml), zinc dust (50 mg) is added and the mixture is heated on a steam bath for 10 minutes. The supernatant liquid is decanted into a test tube and anhydrous sodium acetate (100 mg) and benzoyl chloride (2 drops) are added. The mixture is shaken for 1 minute and N ferric chloride and few drops of dilute hydrochloric acid are added. A red violet to purple colour is appeared.
2. To a 0.1% sample solution (5 ml), add a few drops of silver nitrate solution, no precipitate is produced.
3. Heat the substance (50 mg) with alcoholic potassium hydroxide (2 ml) in a test tube on a water bath for 15 minutes. Acidify with nitric acid and add silver nitrate. A white precipitate of silver chloride is produced.
4. To the substance (20 mg), add sodium hydroxide solution (5 ml) and pyridine (2 ml). Shake well and heat on a water bath. A brownish red colour is developed in the pyridine.

Category : Antibacterial.

PROCAINE PENICILLIN

Syn : Procaine Benzylpenicillin, Procaine Penicillin G.

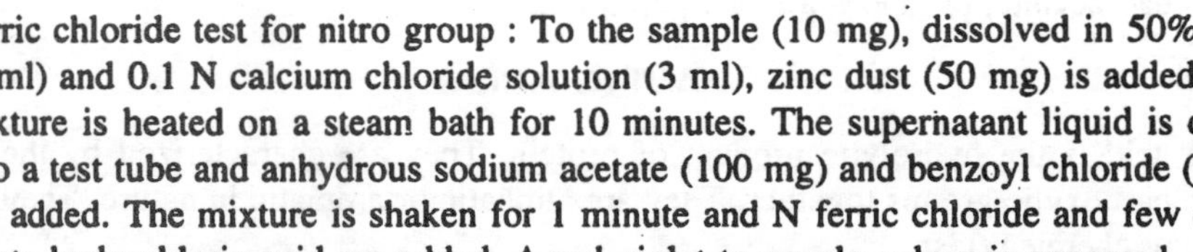

Physical Properties

It is a white crystalline powder; slightly soluble in water.

Chemical Test

Diazotization Test : This test depends upon the presence of the aromatic primary amino group which is a part of the procaine molecule.

Dissolve the substance (0.1 g) in dilute hydrochloric acid with gentle warning, if necessary, cool in an ice and add 1% w/v sodium nitrite solution (4 ml). Pour the solution into a mixture of β—naphthol solution (2 ml) containing sodium acetate (1 g). A bright orange red precipitate is produced (dye formation).

Category : Antibacterial.

GLYCOSIDES

Glycosides are compounds which upon hydrolysis give rise to one or more sugars (glycones) and a compound which is not a sugar (aglycone or genine). Cardioactive glycosides (digitoxin, gitoxin, lanatosides, scillarens, etc.), anthraquinone glycosides (sennosides, barbaloin, cascarosides, etc.), amygdalin, sinigrin, sinalbin and gentiopicroside are the important glycosides of natural origin.

Chemical Tests

1. **Keller-Killiani Test:** To solution of the drug in glacial acetic acid, few drops of ferric chloride and concentrated sulphuric acid are added. A reddish-brown colour is formed at the junction of two layers and the upper layer turns bluish green.
2. **Legal Test:** To a solution of the glycoside in pyridine, sodium nitroprusside and sodium hydroxide solutions are added. A pink to red colour is formed.
3. **Baljet Test:** To an alcoholic solution of the glycoside, sodium picrate reagent is added. A yellow or orange colour in formed in the presence of glycosides.
4. **Borntrager's Test:** A mixture of the glycoside (0.1 g), dilute hydrochloric acid (5 ml) and 5% solution of ferric chloride (5 ml) is boiled for 5 minutes. The solution is cooled, filtered and the filtrate is shaken with benzene. The benzene layer is separated, ammonia solution added to it when a pink colour is formed.
5. **3, 5-Dinitrobenzoic Acid Test:** To an alcoholic solution of the glycoside, few drops of sodium hydroxide solution and 2% solution of 3, 5-dinitrobenzoic acid are added. A pink colour develops.
6. **Fehlings Solution Test:** To an aqueous solution of the glycoside, dilute hydrochloric acid is added and boiled for 10 minutes. The solution is made alkaline by addition of sodium hydroxide solution. Fehlings solutions A and B are added and the reaction mixture heated for 5 minutes. A red precipitate of cuprous oxide is produced.

STEROIDS AND TRITERPENOIDS

Steroids are tetracyclic compounds characterized by the presence of a perhydro–1, 2–cyclo–pentenophenanthrene ring system. The three cyclohexane rings are designated as A, B, C and the cyclopentane ring is the D ring. They are colourless crystalline compounds widely distributed in animals and plants. They possess an alcoholic group and may be saturated or unsaturated. Stigmasterol, β-sitosterol, testosterone, progesterone, cortisone and hydrocortisone are the important steroids.

Triterpenoids have a carbon skeleton based on six isoprene units. They are colourless crystalline, often high melting optically active compounds. The cyclic compounds are the tetracyclic (lanostane, euphane, cycloartane, etc.) or pentacyclic (α-amyrin, β-amyrin, lupane, hopane, glycyrrhizic acid, cucurbitacins, etc.).

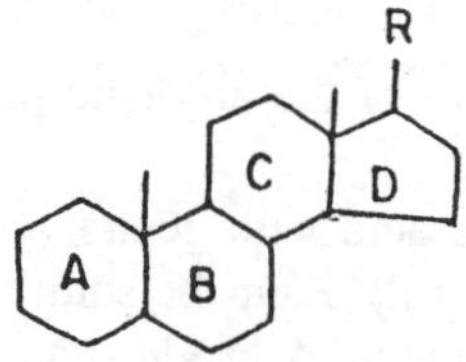

Steroid skeleton

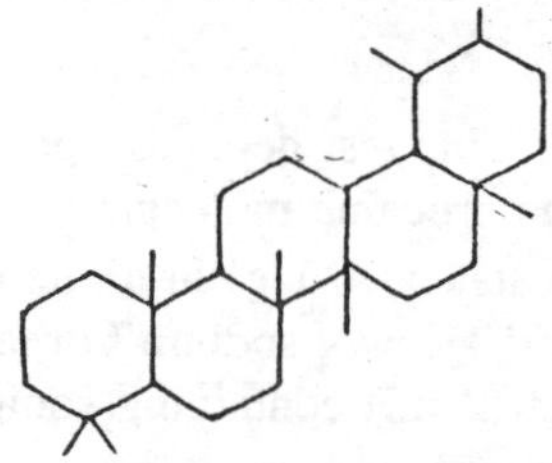

Triterpenoid skelton

Chemical Tests

1. **Liebermann-Burchard Test:** To a chloroform solution of the drug, few drops of acetic anhydride and 1 ml of concentrated sulphuric acid are added. Blue or blood red colour is produced.
2. **Salkovaski Test:** To a chloroform solution of a sterol, concentrated sulphuric acid (2 ml) is added. A yellow ring at the junction is formed which turns red after one minute.
3. **Antimony Trichloride Test:** To a chloroform solution of the drug, a saturated solution of antimony trichloride in chloroform containing 20% acetic anhydride is added and the reaction mixture heated for 10 minutes. A pink colour is developed.
4. **Trichloroacetic Acid Test:** Triterpenes on heating with trichloroacetic acid produces temperature dependent distinct colours.
5. **Tetranitromethane Test:** It gives yellow colour with unsaturated compounds.
6. **Zimmermann Test:** A mixture of alcoholic solution of the compound and m-dinitrobenzene in the presence of an alkali on heating gives violet colour, which faded after dilution for 3-oxo steroids and triterpenes.

SAPONINS

Saponins are highly complex glycosides which are widely distributed in higher plants. The drugs like Quillaia, Sarsaparilla, Senega and Dioscorea have their medicinal properties due to the saponins they contain. Steroidal saponins are less common than the pentacyclic triterpenoid type in plants.

Steroidal saponins have the C_{27}–framework of cholesterol rather than that of the C_{29}–sitosterol. Sugar residue may be linked via single hydroxyl group of the aglycone monodesmoside saponins or more rarely via two hydroxyl groups. Usually the sugars like D-glucose, D-galactose, D-xylose, L-rhamnose and L-arabinose occur in the glycosides.

Diosgenin, tigogenin, smilagenin, yamogenin, hecogenin and gitogenin are the steroidal saponins. Glycyrrhetinic acid is an important pentacyclic triterpenic saponin.

Chemical Tests

1. **Frothing Test:** To an aqueous solution of a saponin, few drops of sodium bicarbonate solution are added and the reaction mixture is shaken. Honey comb-like frothing is formed which persisted for more than 30 minutes.
2. **RBC Haemolysis Test:** Blood (5 ml) is centrifused and the RBC suspended in 10 ml of normal saline. To the suspension (1 ml), the alcoholic solution of glycoside (1 ml) is added. It is shaken when honey comb-like frothing is formed.

RESINS

Resins are solids or semisolid plant exudates of plants. They are almost plant products; shellac is an exception which is an insect secretion. Chemically, they are complex mixtures of compounds like aliphatic alcohols, resin acids, phenols, esters and terpenes.

Physical Properties

Usually resins are amorphonus, brittle, transluscent, hard solids. On heating they are softened and then melt. They are practically insoluble in water but dissolve in alcohol, ether and chloroform. Varnish—like film is formed on evaporation of the solvent. They produce smoky flame on burning.

Chemical Tests

1. To an alcoholic solution, distilled water is added. A turbidity is formed.
2. To an alcoholic solution, acetone (3 ml) and concentrated hydrochloric acid (3 ml) are added and the reaction mixture is heated for 30 minutes. A pink colour is developed.

FLAVONOIDS

Flavonoids contains fifteen carbon atoms in their basic nucleus and these are arranged in a $C_6 - C_3 - C_6$ configuration, that is, two aromatic rings liked by a three carbon unit which may or may not form a third ring. They occur both in the free state and as glycosides and are the largest group of naturally occurring phenols. They are commonly found as flavonoids O-glycosides in which one or more of the flavonoid hydroxyl groups is bound to a sugar(s). Sugars may also be C-linked to the flavonoid. In this case they are attached directly to the benzene nucleus by a carbon-carbon bond which is acid resistant. Biflavonoids are flavonoid dimers. The glycosides are generally soluble in water and alcohol, but insoluble in organic solvents; the genins are only sparingly soluble in water but are soluble in ether. Flavonoids dissolve in alkalies, giving yellow solutions which on the addition of acid become colourless.

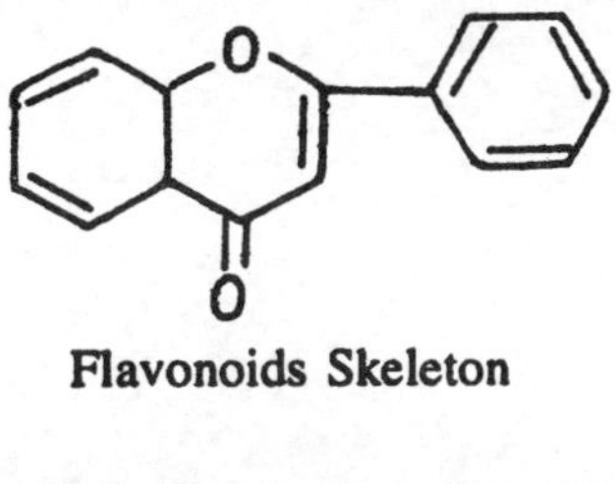

Flavonoids Skeleton

Chemical Tests

1. **Ammonia Test:** A filter paper dipped in an alcoholic solution of the flavonoid is exposed to vapours of ammonia solution. A yellow colour is formed.
2. **Shinoda Test:** To an alcoholic solution of the extract, few chips of magnesium turnings and dilute hydrochloric acid (2 ml) are added. A red colour is produced. If magnesium in replaced by zinc, only dihydroflavonols gives deep red to magneta colour.
3. **Vanillin- HCl Test:** To the alcoholic solution of a flavonoid, vanillin-hydrochloric reagent is added. A pink colour is formed.

FIXED OILS AND FATS

Fixed oils and fats are esters of glycerol with higher long-chain fattly acids such as palmitic, stearic, oleic and linoleic acids. The fatty acids may be saturated (e.g. palmitic acid, stearic acid) or unsaturated (e.g. oleic acid), but usually they contain unbranched carbon chains and have an even number of carbon atoms.

Physical Characters.

Fats and oils are greasy substances and are lighter than water. They are insoluble in water, sparingly soluble in alcohol, and freely soluble in ether, chloroform and benzene. Their specific gravity is less than water. They cannot be distilled and on heating they are decomposed to form acraldehyde.

Chemical Tests

1. **Spot Test:** A drop of petroleum ether solution of an oil or fat is put on a filter paper piece and allowed to evaporate. Oily spot is formed.
2. **Saponification Test:** A mixture of an oil or fat (1 g), 0.5 N alcoholic potassium hydroxide solution (5 ml) and 1 drop of phenolphthalein solution is neutralized on heating and a soap is formed.
3. **Bromine Water Test:** To carbon tetrachloride solution of the oil or fat, bromine water (2 ml) is added and shaken. Decolourization of the bromine water indicated unsaturation in the molecule.

VOLATILE OILS

1. Volatile oils have characteristic preasant odour.
2. A spot of the volatile oil on a filter paper piece is evaporated with 24 hours.

Volatile or essential oils are mono- and sesquiterpenes obtained from certain plant parts. They are colourless liquids and are lighter than water. They possess distinct odours, have high refractive indices, generally are optically active and immiscible with water. Volatile oils are freely soluble in ether, alcohol, chloroform, acetone, etc.

13

Organic Preparations

1. Preparation of Aspirin from Salicylic Acid

Requirements :

Salicylic acid	=	10 g
Acetic anhydride	=	14 ml
Conc. H_2SO_4	=	2 ml

Chemical Reaction :

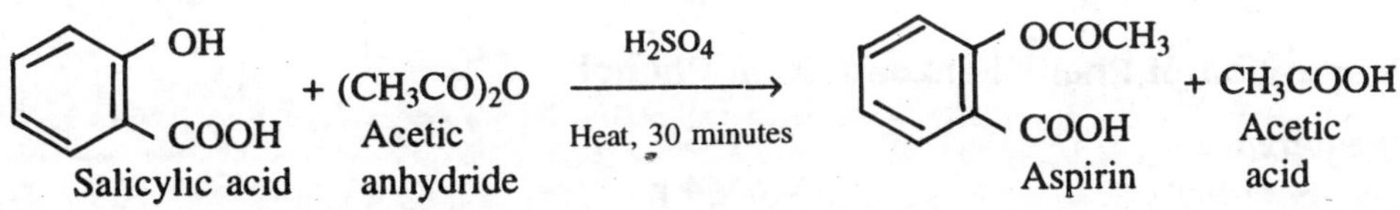

Procedure : Take salicylic acid (10 g), acetic anhydride (14 ml) and concentrated suphuric acid (2 ml) and warm the reaction mixture for half an hour at 50-60° with frequent stirring. Pour down the contents into cold water (150 ml) with occasional stirring and filter off the crude aspirin. For recrystallization, dissolve the product in alcohol (30 ml) and pour the solution into warm water (75 ml). If a solid separates, warm the mixture to dissolve the solid. The clear solution is allowed to cool slowly to get needle shaped crystals of aspirin, m.p. 136—137°, yield 13 g.

2. Preparation of Acetanilide from Aniline

Requirements:

Aniline	=	20 ml
Acetic anhydride	=	20 ml
Glacial acetic acid	=	20 ml

Chemical Reaction

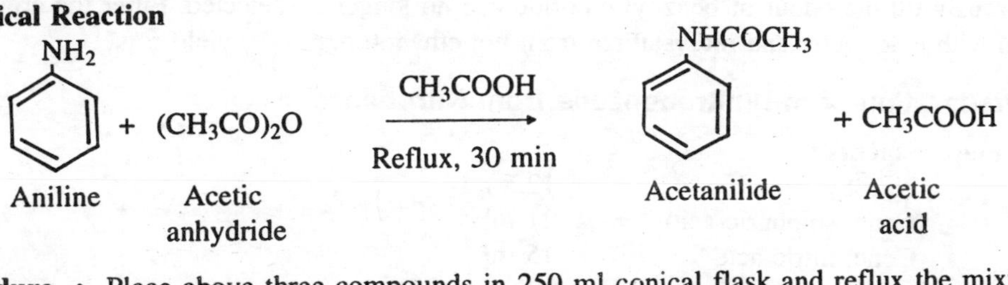

Procedure : Place above three compounds in 250 ml conical flask and reflux the mixture for 30 minutes with frequent shaking. Pour down the contents into ice-cold water with constant stirring. Filter the crude acetanilide, wash with cold water and recrystallize from boiling water along with small quantity of methylated spirit; m.p. 114°, yield 21 g .

3. Preparation of Benzanilide from Aniline

Requirement:

Aniline	=	5 ml
Benzoyl chloride	=	7 ml
10 % sodium hydroxide	=	45 ml

Chemical Reaction:

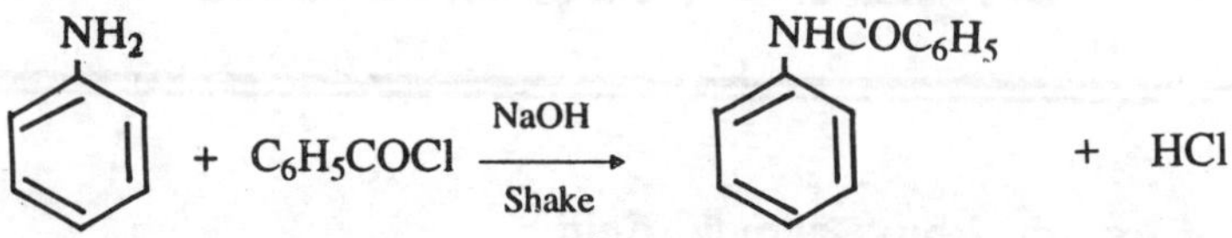

Aniline — Benzoyl chloride — Benzanilide

Procedure : Place aniline (5 ml), 10 % sodium hydroxide solution (45 ml) in 250 ml conical flask and then add slowly benzoyl chloride (7 ml) with vigorous shaking. Cork the flask and shake for further 15 minutes or till the odour of benzoyl chloride can no longer be detected. Dilute the reaction mixture with cold water (100 ml). Filter off the crude benzanilide with suction on a buchner funnel, wash with cold water and recrystallize from hot alcohol, m.p. 162°, yield 9 g.

4. Preparation of Phenylbenzoate from Phenol

Requirement:

Phenol	=	4 g
Benzoyl chloride	=	8 ml
10 % Sodium hydroxide	=	60 ml

Chemical Reaction:

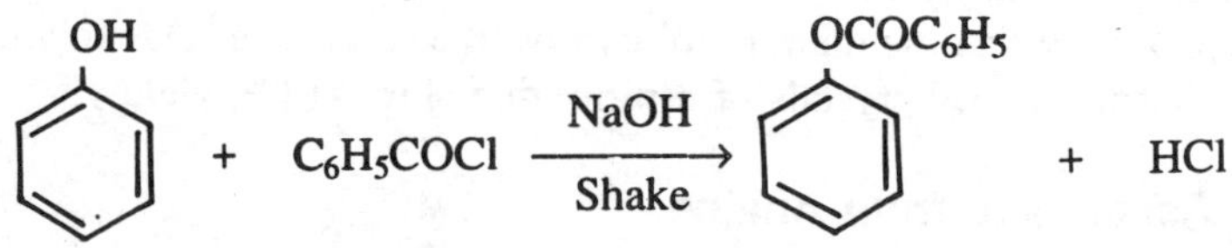

Phenol — Benzoyl chloride — phenylbenzoate

Procedure : Add phenol (4 ml) to 10 % sodium hydroxide solution (60 ml) in 250 ml conical flask. Add benzoyl chloride (8 ml) slowly with constant shaking. Cork the flask and shake it vigorously till the odour of benzoyl chloride can no longer be detected. Filter the crude product, wash with cold water and recrystallize from hot ethanol, m.p. 69°, yield 6 g.

5. Preparation of m-Dinitrobenzene from Nitrobenzene

Requirements :

Nitrobenzene	=	12.5 ml
Conc. sulphuric acid	=	21 ml
Conc. nitric acid	=	15 ml

Chemical Reaction :

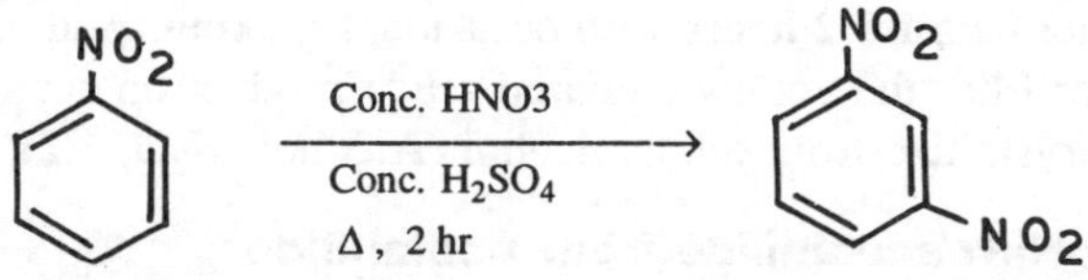

Nitrobenzene m—Dinitrobenzene

Procedure : Place concentrated sulphuric acid (21 ml) and concentrated nitric acid (15 ml) in 250 ml round bottomed flask containing few small pieces of unglazed porcelain to prevent bumping. Attach reflux condenser and add slowly nitrobenzene in a portion of 2-3 ml with shaking. Cool the mixture and then pour it into ice cold water with stirring. Filter the crude m—dinitrobenzene with suction, wash with cold water and recrystallize from hot methylated (or rectified) spirit to obtain yellow crystalline substance, m.p. 90°, yield 15 g.

6. Preparation of 2, 4, 6-Tribromoaniline from Aniline

Requirements :

Aniline	=	20 ml
Glacial acetic acid	=	20 ml.
Bromine in glacial acetic acid	=	8.4 ml in 20 ml of glacial acetic acid

Chemical Reaction

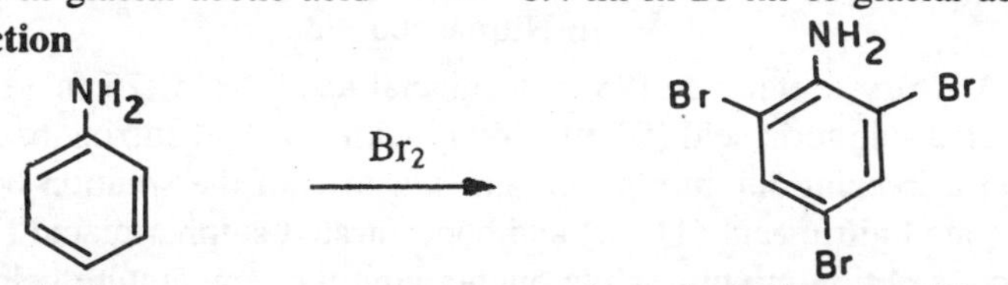

Aniline 2, 4, 6—Tribromoaniline

Procedure : Take aniline (5 ml) and glacial acetic acid (20 ml) in a 250 ml conical flask. Add to it dropwise bromine (8.4 ml) , dissolve in glacial acetic acid (20 ml) with constant stirring while keeping the flask in an ice bath. A solid mass so obtained is filtered, washed with cold water and recrystallized from dilute alcohol to obtain colourless crystals, m.p. 120°C, yield 10 g.

7. Preparation of Picric Acid (2,4,6-Trinitrophenol) from Phenol

Requirements :

Phenol	=	10 g
Conc. HNO_3	=	38 ml
Conc. H_2SO_4	=	12.5 ml

Chemical Reaction :

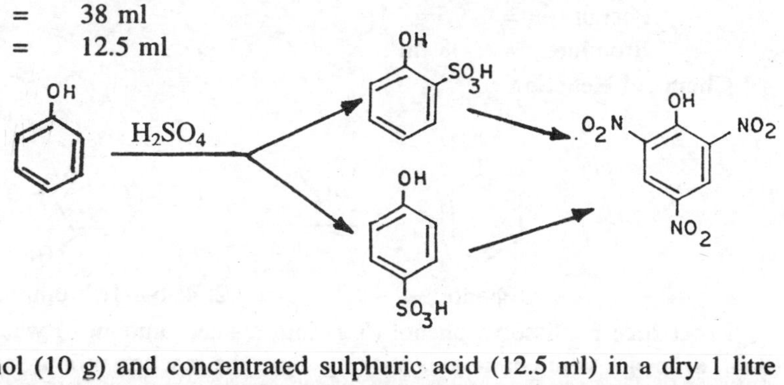

Procedure : Take phenol (10 g) and concentrated sulphuric acid (12.5 ml) in a dry 1 litre flat bottomed flask and heat the mixture on a water bath for 30 minutes with frequent shaking to form the o- and p-phenolsulphonic acid. Cool the flask in an ice bath and add concentrated nitric acid (38 ml) dropwise with constant shaking (this step should be carried in funning cupboard).

Allow the reaction mixture to stand for sometime and when evolution of red fumes are stopped, heat the flask on a water bath for 2 hours with occasional shaking. Add cold water (100 ml), chill thoroughly in ice water filter the yellow coloured crude product on suction, wash with water till free from acid and recrystallize from dilute alcohol (Alcohol: H_2O, 1:2), m.p. 122°, yield 16 g.

8. Preparation of p-Nitroacetanilide from Acetanilide

Requirements :

Acetanilide	=	25 g
Glacial acetic acid	=	10 ml
Conc. H_2SO_4	=	50 ml
Conc. HNO_3	=	11 ml

Chemical Reaction:

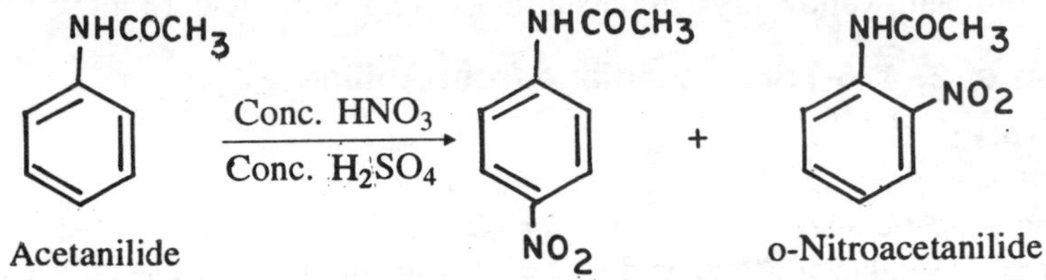

p-Nitroacetanilide

Procedure : Add dry acetanilide (25 g) to glacial acetic acid (25 ml) in a beaker and then introduce concentrated sulphuric acid (50 ml) slowly with constant stirring to obtain clear solution. Place the beaker in a freezing mixture of ice and salt to cool the solution below 5°. Add a cold mixture of concentrated nitric acid (11 ml) and concentrated sulphuric acid (7 ml) dropwise with constant stirring to a reaction mixture while maintaining the temperature below 5°. After adding all the mixed acid, remove the beaker from the freezing mixture and keep it for 1 hour at room temperature. Pour the reaction mixture into an ice cold water (30 ml) to obtain the crude product of nitroacetanilide. Filter it on suction, wash with cold water till free from acid and recrystallize the pale yellow product from alcohol to get colourless crystalline solid, m.p. 214°, yield 20 g.

Note : o-Nitroacetanilide remains in the filtrate due to its more solubility in H_2O.

9. Preparation of 2, 4, 6-Tribromophenol from Phenol

Requirement :

Phenol	=	5 g
Bromine	=	8 ml

Chemical Reaction :

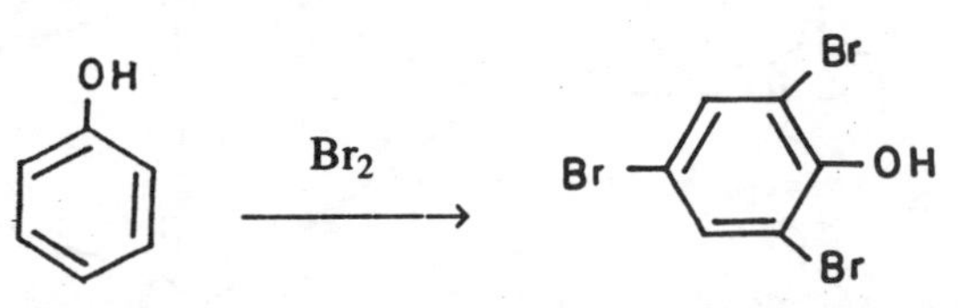

Phenol 2, 4, 6—Tribromophenol

Procedure : Dissolve phenol (5 g) into a small amount of water and add bromine solution (8 ml) dropwise with continuous shaking. Pour the reaction mixture into ice cold water. Filter the crude product, wash with water and recrystallize with dilute alcohol to obtain colourless crystalline material, m.p. 93°, yield 12 g.

10. Preparation of p-Bromoacetanilide from Acetanilide

Requirement :

Acetanilide	=	13.5 g
Glacial acetic acid	=	70 ml
Bromine	=	5.5 ml
Sodium bisulphite	=	sufficient quantity

Chemical Reaction :

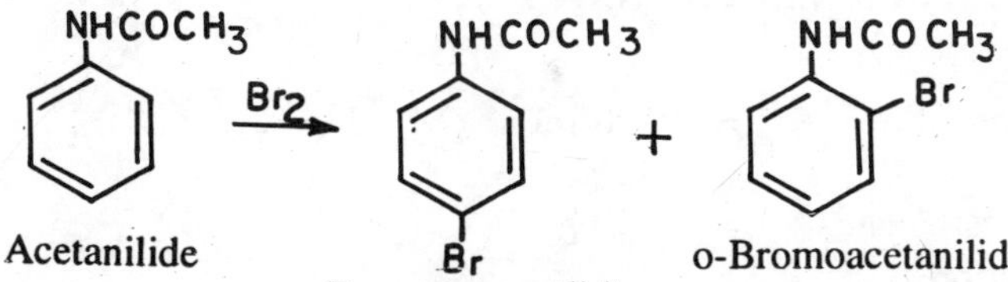

Acetanilide p-Bromoacetanilide o-Bromoacetanilide

Procedure : Dissolve acetanilide (13.5 g) in glacial acetic acid (45 ml) in 250 ml conical flask. Add dropwise by burette, bromine (5.5 ml) dissolved in glacial acetic acid (25 ml) with constant shaking. (Precaution : reaction should be carried out in fuming cupboard). Allow to stand the orange coloured reaction mixture at room temperature for half an hour and then pour the contents into cold water. Stir well and add sufficient sodium bisulphite to discharge orange colour which is due to slight brown colour of bromine. Filter the crude product, wash with cold water and recrystallize with dilute alcohol to obtain white crystalline compound, m.p. 167°, yield 18 g.

Note : o-Bromoacetanilide remains in the alcoholic solution during crystallization due to its high solubility.

11 Preparation of p-Bromobenzanilide from Benzanilide

Requirement :

Benzanilide	=	2 gm
Glacial acetic acid	=	30 ml
Bromine	=	2 ml

Chemical Reaction :

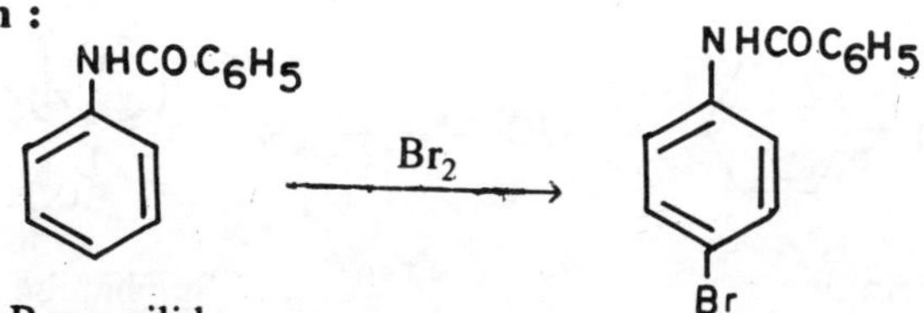

Benzanilide p-Bromobenzanilide

Procedure : Same as in p-Bromoacetainilide

12. Preparation of Phthalimide form Phthalic anhydride

Requirement :

Phthalic anhydride	=	10 g
Urea	=	2 g

Chemical Reaction:

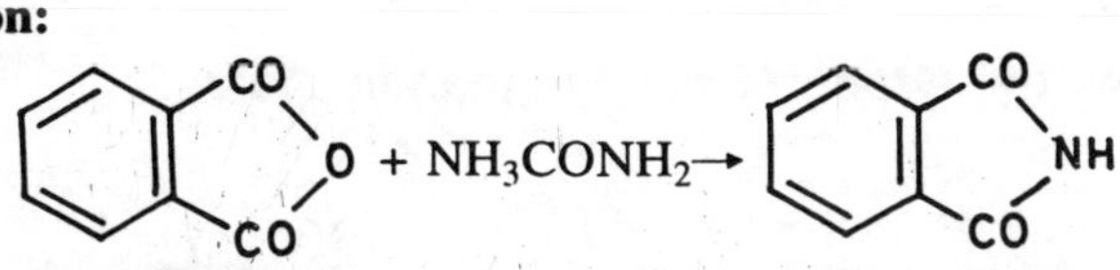

Phthalic anhydride Urea Phthalimide

Procedure : Mix phthalic anhydride (10 g) and urea (2 g) in a 250 ml round bottom flask. Heat the flask on an oil bath or heating mantle at 130—135° till the contents melt, froth up and become solid. Remove the flame beneath the bath and allow to cool. Add water (about 50 ml) to disintegrate the solid. Filter the crude product, wash with little water and recrystallize from alcohol to obtain white product, melting point 232°, yield 8 g.

Note : Concentrated ammonia solution can be used in place of urea.

13. Preparation of Iodoform from Ethyl Alcohol

Requirement :

Ethyl alcohol	=	20 ml
Iodine	=	3 g
Sodium carbonate	=	40 g

Chemical Reaction :

$$C_2H_5OH + 4I_2 + 3Na_2CO_3 \rightarrow CHI_3 + 5NaI + HCOONa + CO_2 + 2H_2O$$

Ethyl alcohol Iodoform

Procedure: Take ethyl alcohol (20 ml), sodium carbonate (40g) and water (20 ml) in 500 ml round bottomed flask. Heat the flask to about 70-80° on a water bath. To the warm solution, add small amount of iodine at a time with constant shaking. Add more iodine so that the reaction product should have a pale yellow colour. Add dropwise a dilute solution of sodium hydroxide if any brown colour of iodine persists. Filter the crude iodoform, wash with cold water and recrystallize from hot ethanol to obtain the yellow crystals, m.p. 119°, yield 12 g.

14. Preparation of Sulphanilic Acid from Aniline

Requirement :

Aniline	=	20 ml
Conc. H_2SO_4	=	40 ml

Chemical Reaction :

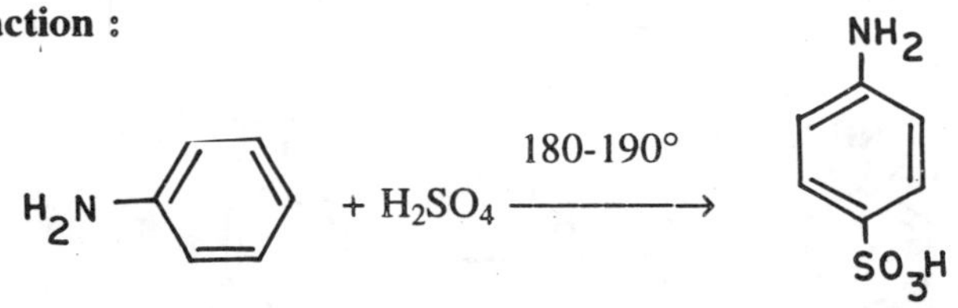

Aniline Sulphanilic acid

Procedure : Add concentrated sulphuric acid (40 ml) dropwise with gentle shaking to aniline (20 ml) in a 250 ml conical flask. Keep the flask cool by occasionally immersing in cold water. Heat the flak on an oil bath at 180-190° for 5 hours (Precaution : Reaction should be carried out in fuming cupboard. Completion of the reaction can be checked by dissolving the reaction mixture (2 ml) in 2 N sodium hydroxide (3 ml) without leaving the solution cloudy.

Cool the contents and pour them carefully into ice-cold water. The crude sulphanilic acid is filtered off on Buchner funnel, wash well with cold water and recrystallized from boiling distilled water to obtain shining white crystals, m.p. 300°(decomposes), yield 20 g.

15. Preparation of Methyl Orange from Sulphanilic Acid

Requirement :

Sulphanilic acid	=	10.5 g

Anhydrous sodium carbonate	=	3 g
Sodium nitrate	=	3.5 g
Dimethyl aniline	=	6.5 ml
Sodium chloride	=	10 g
20 % NaOH solution	=	3.5 ml
Conc. HCl	=	10.5 ml

Chemical Reaction :

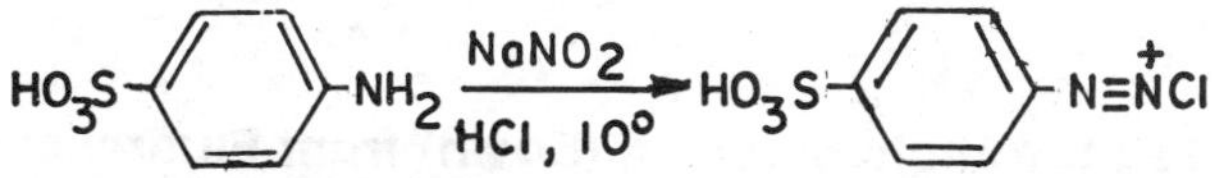

Sulphanilic acid

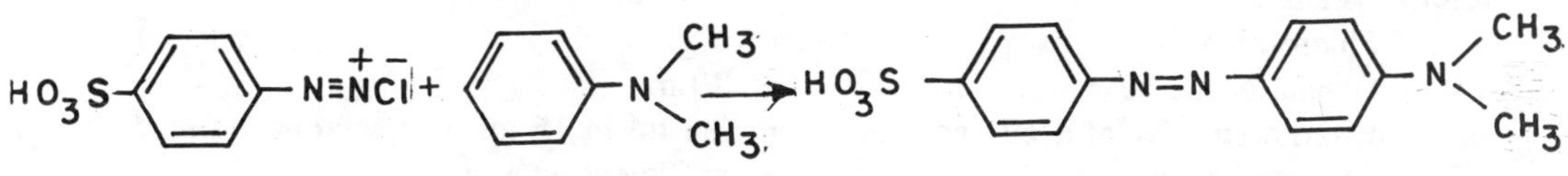

Dimethyl aniline methyl orange.

Procedure : Sulphanilic acid, (10.5 g) and sodium carbonate (3 g) are dissolved in water (about 100 ml) by gentle warning. Cool the solution below 10° and add sodium nitrite (3.5 g) dissolved in water (10 ml). Pour the resulting solution slowly with stirring into a 500 ml beaker containing concentrated hydrochloric acid (10.5 ml) while maintaining the temperature below 10°. Fine crystals of diazobenzene sulphonate separate out. Add dimethyl aniline (6.5 ml) in glacial acetic acid (3 ml) with vigorous stirring to a suspension of diazobenzene sulphonate. Allow to stand for 10 minutes, the red methyl orange will gradually separate. Add 20 % sodium hydroxide solution (35 ml) with stirring to separate out the sodium salt of methyl orange. Warm the solution to about 80°C and add sodium chloride (10 g) (helps in the separation of methyl orange). Shake, cool the mixture in an ice bath and filter the methyl orange under very gentle pressure. Wash the crude product with cold water and recrystallize from boiling water to obtain orange red crystals, yield 13 g.

16. Preparation of Fluorescein from Phthalic Anhydride

Requirements :

Phthalic anhydride	=	7.5 gms
Resorcinol	=	12 gms
Anhydrous zinc chloride	=	5 gm
Conc. hydrochloric acid	=	8 ml

Chemical Reaction :

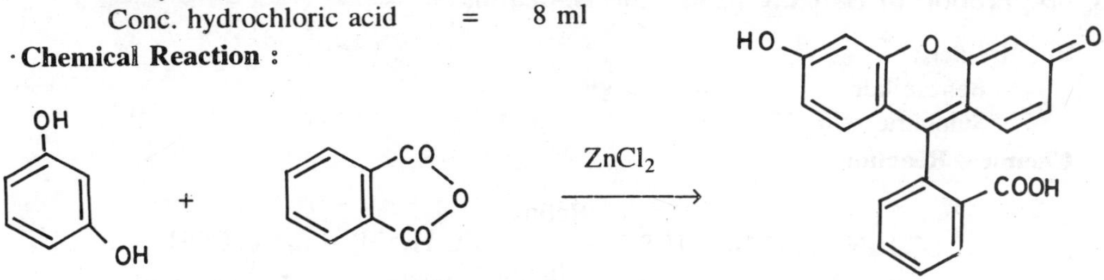

Resorcinol Phthalic anhydride Fluorescein

Procedure : Grind phthalic anhydride (7.5 g) and resorcinol (12 g) in a mortar and then transfer to 500 ml round bottom flask. Heat the contents to 180° on an oil bath. While oil bath is being heated, weigh rapidly anhydrous zinc chloride (5 g). Powder it and then transfer in a stopper bottle. Add zinc chloride in small portion from the stoppered bottle to the flask with stirring the mixture. Continue heating at 180-190° while stirring at interval of 2-3 minutes until it solidifies completely (about 1 hour is required). Cool the flask, add water (about 150 ml) and concentrated hydrochloric acid (8 ml). Again heat the solution to boiling with frequent stirring. Continue boiling till whole zinc salt is dissolved. Filter the insoluble residue of fluorescein on suction pump, grind it with water, filter again and dry at 100°. It may be purified by dissolving it in dilute sodium hydroxide, filtering if necessary, precipitating with dilute hydrochloric acid, re-filtering, washing and drying, yield 12 g.

17. Preparation of Tetrabromofluorescein (Eosin) from Fluoreseein.

Requirement :

Fluorescein	=	5 g
Glacial acetic acid	=	20 ml
Bromine in glacial acetic acid	=	3.8 ml in 15 ml of glacial acetic acid
Saturated sodium bisulphite solution	=	sufficient quantity.

Chemical Reaction :

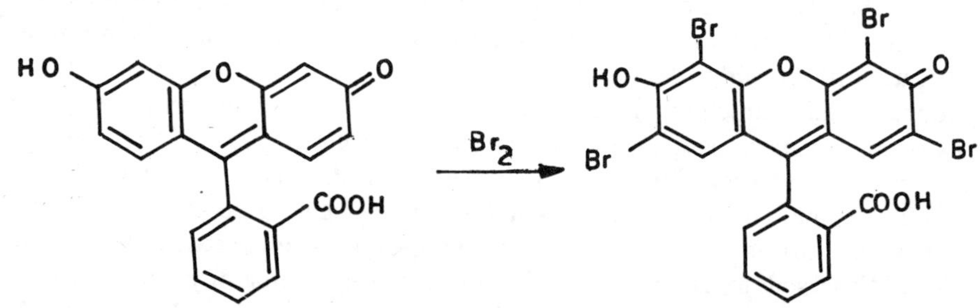

Fluorescein Eosin (Tetrabromo fluorescein)

Procedure : Add powdered fluorescein (5 g) to glacial acetic acid (20 ml) in 100 ml conical flask. Add dropwise a solution of bromine solution (3.8 ml) dissolved in glacial acetic acid (15 ml) by means of a separating funnel or burette. Heat the mixture on a water bath for one hour. Cool the flask and the content are poured into cold water (300 ml) with stirring. If colour of bromine persists, a few drops of sodium bisulphite solution may be added. Filter the crude eosin on suction pump, wash with water and dry. yield 8 g.

18. Preparation of Benzoic Acid from Benzanilide

Requirement :

Benzanilide	=	5 gm
Sulphuric acid (70 %)	=	50 ml

Chemical Reaction :

$$\underset{\text{Benzanilide}}{C_6H_5NHCOC_6H_5} + H_2SO_4 \xrightarrow[\text{30 min}]{\text{Reflux}} \underset{\text{Aniline}}{C_6H_5NH_2} + \underset{\text{Benzoic acid}}{C_6H_5COOH}$$

Procedure : Take benzanilide (5 g) and 70 % sulphuric acid (20 ml) in 100 ml conical flask. Reflux the mixture for half an hour. Remove the flame beneath the flask, pour hot water (60 ml) through reflux condensor and cool the flask in ice water. Filter the benzoic acid, wash with water and recrystallize from boiling water, m.p. 121°, yield 5 g.

Aniline can be recovered by making the filtrate alkaline with 10 % NaOH solution followed by extraction with ether.

19. Preparation of Glucosazone from Glucose

Requirements :

Glucose	=	4 g
Phenylhydrazinc hydrochloride	=	10 g
Sodium acetate	=	10 g

Chemical Reaction :

$$
\begin{array}{lcl}
CHO & & CH = N - NHC_6H_5 \\
| & & | \\
CHOH \quad + \quad 3C_6H_5NHNH_2 & \longrightarrow & C = N\,.\,NHC_6H_5 \\
| & & | \\
(CH_2OH)_3 & & (CHOH)_3 \\
| & & | \\
CH_2OH & & CH_2OH \\
\text{Glucose} & & \text{Glucosazone}
\end{array}
$$

Procedure : Take glucose (4 g), phenylhydrazine hydrochloride (10 g) and sodium acetate (10 g) in a beaker. Add to it water (100 ml) and heat the content for half an hour on water bath. Cool the beaker in an ice bath, yellow crystals of gulcosazone precipitate out. Filter the crude product, wash with cold water and recrystallize it from alcohol, yield 5 g, m.p. 205°

20. Preparation of 2, 2 bis (p-Chlorophenyl)-1, 1, 1-Trichloroethane (D.D.T.).

Requirements :

Chloralhydrate	=	17 g
Chlorobenzene	=	23 ml
Conc. sulphuricacid	=	180 ml

Chemical Reaction:

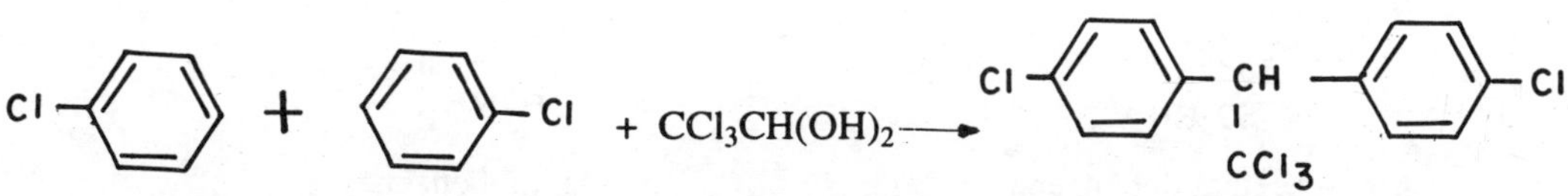

Chlorobenzene Chloral hydrate D.D.T

Procedure : Place chloral hydrate (17 g) and chlorobenzene (23 ml) in 500 ml stoppered flask and warm on a water bath with occasional shaking until all the crystals are dissolved. Cool the flask, add concentrated sulphuric acid (180 ml) slowly and shake mechanically for 1.5 hours and then allow to stand for 15 minutes. Pour the contents slowly into cold water (500 ml) with constant stirring. Filter the crude D.D.T. through sintered glass funnel, wash with water and then add the solids into solution of 2 % sodium carbonate or 4% sodium bicarbonate. Filter again and wash with water until filtrate is neutral to litmus. Transfer the residue in a mortar containing ethyl alcohol (100 ml) and triturate with pestle for 10 minutes. Filter, wash the residue with a small amount of alcohol and dry at 70° in a steam oven, yield 15 g, m.p. 107°. It may be recrystallized from propyl alcohol to obtain pure compound m.p. 108°.

21. Preparation of Sulphanilamide from Acetanilide

Requirements :

Acetanilide	=	20 g
Chlorosulphonic acid	=	50 ml
Strong ammonia solution	=	70 ml
Hydrochloric acid		Sufficient
Sodium bicarbonate		quantity

Chemical Reaction :

There are three steps of reactions

First steps:

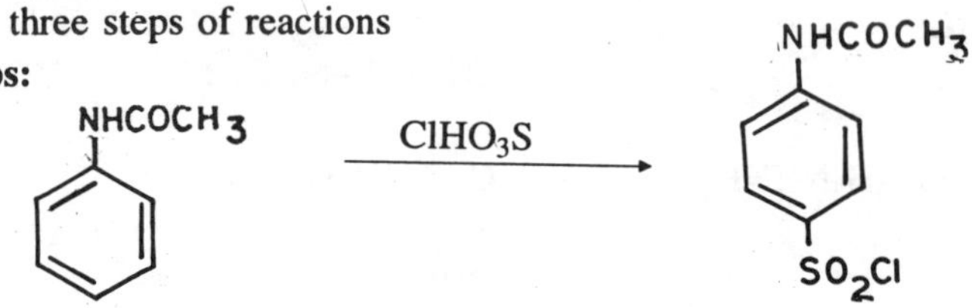

Acetanilide — p–Acetamidobenzene sulphonyl chloride

Second Step:

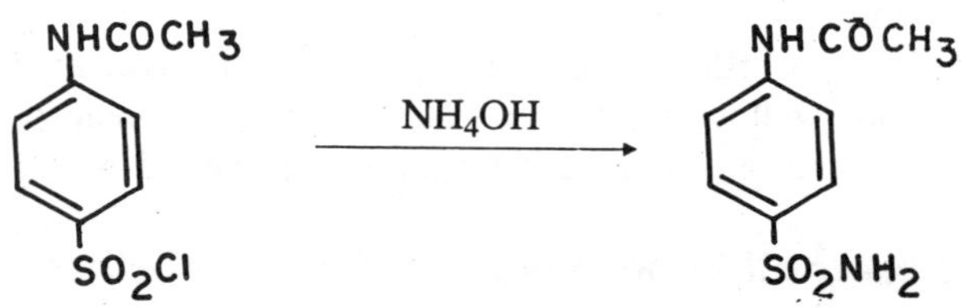

p—Acetamidobenzene sulphon amide

Third Step:

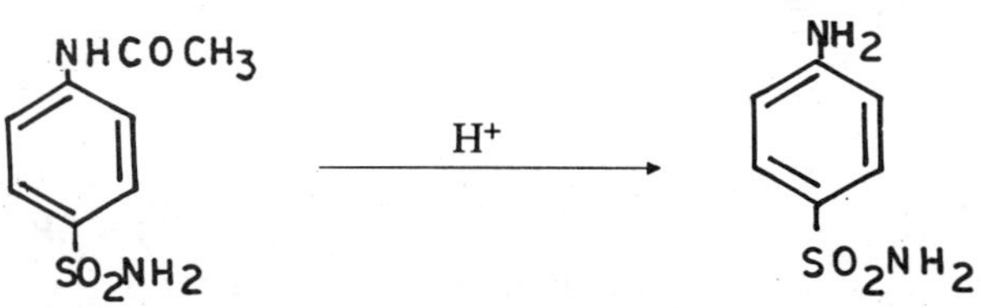

p—Acetamidobenzene sulphonamide — p—Aminobenzene sulphonamide

Procedure

Step-I : Preparation of p–Acetamidobenzene sulphonyl chloride

Take dry acetanilide (20 g) in 500 ml two mouth round bottom flask. The flask is fitted with dropping funnel and a reflux condensor. Attach a gas trap device to the top of the condensor (Fig. 13.1). Place chlorosulphonic acid (50 ml) in a dropping funnel and fix a calcium chloride guard tube to it. Add chlorosulphonic acid in small portions to the acetanilide with occasional shaking to ensure thorough mixing.

Heat the mixture for 1 hour in order to complete the reaction. Allow to cool and pour the oily mixture into ice-cold water. Filter the crude product on suction pump, wash with cold water and press well to obtain the dry product of p-acetamidobenzene sulphonyl chloride.

Note : Chlorosulphuric acid must be handled with great care, it is very corrosive to the skin and to clothing and reacts with water with violence.

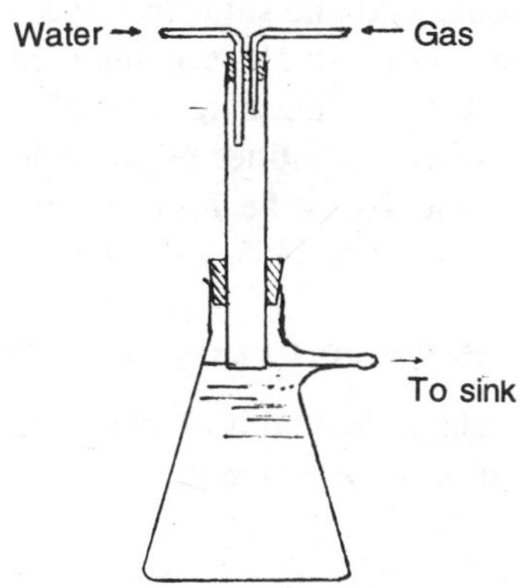

Fig. 13.1. Gas Absorption Trap

Step-II : Preparation of p-Acetamidosulphonamide

Add a mixture of strong ammonia solution (70 ml) and water (70 ml) to a crude p-acetamidobenzene sulphonyl chloride in a 500 ml flask. Heat the contents with occasional shaking for about 15 minutes to just below the boiling point.

Cool the suspension in ice and then add dilute sulphuric acid until the mixture is just acidic to Congo red paper (pH 2-3). Filter the crude p-acetamidobenzene sulphonamide, wash it with cold water and dry in air, yield 18 g.

Step-III : Preparation of p-Aminobenzene sulphonamide :

Add the crude p-acetamidobenzene suphonamide to a mixture of concentrated hydrochloric acid (10 ml) and water (30 ml). Boil the mixture gently under reflux for 30–45 minutes. The solution when cooled to room temperature, should not deposit the solid amide; if a solid separates, heat further for a short period. Heat the solution to boiling with decolourizing carbon (2 g) for 15 minutes, filter and to the filtrate, cautiously add sufficient sodium bicarbonate in portions with stirring until the solution becomes neutral. Cool the solution, filter the crude sulphanilamide with suction and dry. Then crude product is recrystallized from water or from alcohol to obtain pure product, m.p. 163—164°, yield 15 g.

22. Isolation of Caffeine (1, 3, 7—Trimethylxanthine)

Caffeine is a xanthine base found in tea leaves to the extent of 5% and so it is extracted from tea leaves.

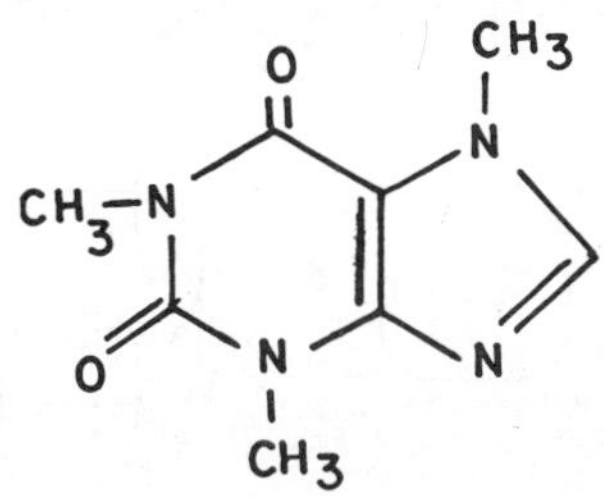

Caffeine

Requirement :

Tea leaves	= 100 g
Basic lead acetate	= 300 ml
Dilute H_2SO_4 solution.	= Sufficient quantity.
Chloroform	= 150
Decolourizing carbon	= 1 g.

Procedure : Boil dry tea leaves (100 g) with water for half an hour. Filter it through muslin cloth and add to the filtrate with gentle warming, a sufficient quantity of 10% basic lead acetate solution until precipitation of tannins is completed. Filter the hot solution and add sufficient amount of dilute sulphuric acid to the filtrate to precipitate excess of lead acetate as insoluble lead sulphate. Filter off lead sulphate and the filtrate is concentrated by evaporation to about 300 ml. Add the decolourizing carbon (1 g), boil the mixture and filter. The filtrate is extracted with three successive quantities of chloroform (3 × 50 ml). The combined chloroform extract is evaporated to dryness and the residue obtained is recrystallized from water to obtain the silky needles of caffeine, m.p. 235°, yield 1 g.

23. Isolation of Eugenol from Cinnamon Leaf Oil

Cinnamon leaf oil is obtained from the leaves of *Cinnamonum zeylanicum* (Lauraceae). It contains about 85% of eugenol.

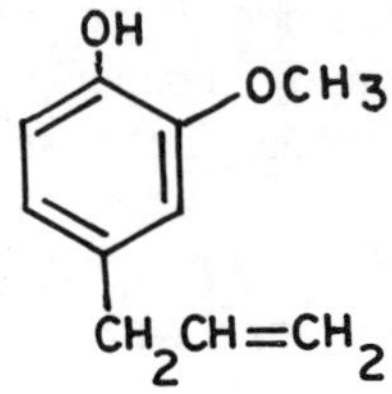

Requirements:

Volatile oil	= 10 ml
Solvant ether	= 250 ml
Potassium hydroxide (10%)	= 300 ml

Procedure : Dissolve volatile oil (10 ml) in solvent ether (100 ml) and shake with 10% potassium hydroxide solution (3 × 100 ml). Regenerate eugenol by acidifying the aqueous layer with excess of sulphuric acid and extracting the acidified layer with solvent ether (3 × 50 ml). Distil off the solvent slowly and dry the eugenol in a desiccator.

24. Isolation of Pectin from Orange Peels

Pectin in a yellowish white powder with mucilaginous taste. Solution of pection (1 g) in hot water (9 ml) forms a stiff jelly on cooling.

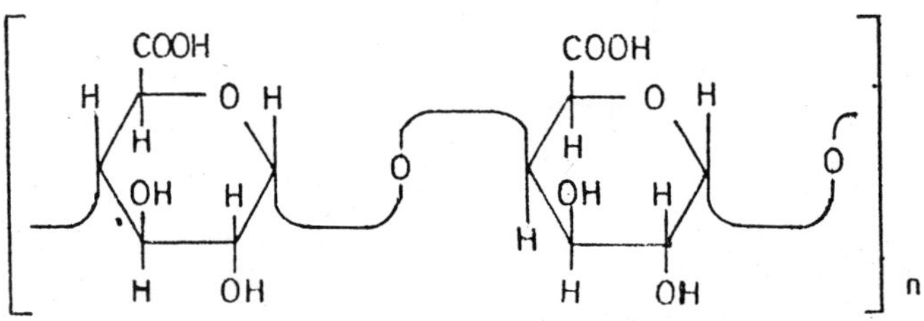

Requirements

Orange peel	= 250 ml
Acetone	= Sufficient amount
Demineralized water	= 1 litre
Citric acid	= Sufficient amount

Procedure: Small pieces of peels (250 g) are washed thoroughly with water and immerse in demineralized water (1 litre). Adjust the pH to 4.5 with citric acid. Heat the contents at about 90° with stirring for 1 hour. Add filter aid and filter rapid the hot solution. Cool the filtrate and pour it slowly into 3 volumes of acetone or isopropanol. Stir the solution thoroughly for the precipitation of pection. Filter through nylon sieve. Wash the residue several times with acetone or isopropanol (70%) to free it from acidic ions. Dry the product in vacuum. The yield is 4-5%.

25. Isolation of Aloin from Aloe

Aloe contains up to 30% aloin which is a mixture of barbaloin, isobarbaloin and β-barbaloin.

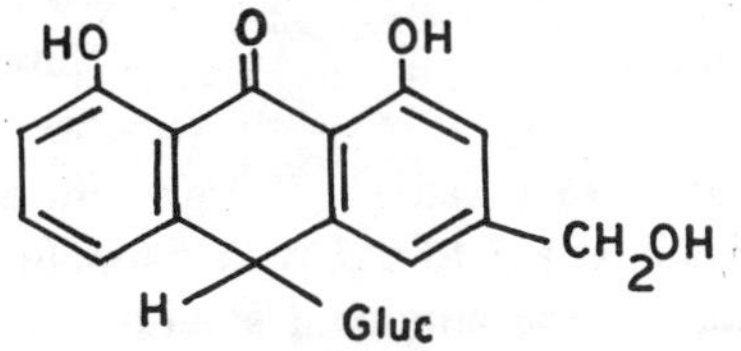

Aloin

Requirements:

Aloe	= 100 g
Water	= 1 litre
Sulphuric acid	= Sufficient amount
Ammonia solution	= Sufficient amount
Ethanol (50%)	= 50 ml

Procedure: Dissolve powdered aloe (100 g) in boiling water (1 litre), stir and filter. Acidify the filtrate with sulphuric acid to precipitate the resinous mass. Separate the precipitate by vacuum filtration and discard. Neutralize the filtrate with ammonia, and allow to stand overnight. The crystalline product is filtered and recrystallized from 50% ethanol. The yield is 10-15%.

26. Isolation of Starch from Potatoes

Starch $(C_6H_{10}O_5)_n$ is present in different parts of a plant in the form of grains. It consists of amylopectin and amylose.

Requirements:

Potatoes	= 500 g
Water	= Sufficient amount.

Procedure: Wash potatoes (500 g) thoroughly with water the remove any soil particles. Prepare a fine slurry with water in a blender. Pass the slurry through a sieve with shaking to remove all debris and other impurities. Allow the milky liquid to settle down. Decent the supernatant liquid. Wash starch 2-3 times with water. Centrifuge in an oven at low temperature and grind. The yield of starch is about 10%. It gives blue colour with iodine solution.

27. Isolation of Solanine from Potato

Solanine is a steroidal glycoalkaloid present in potato plant.

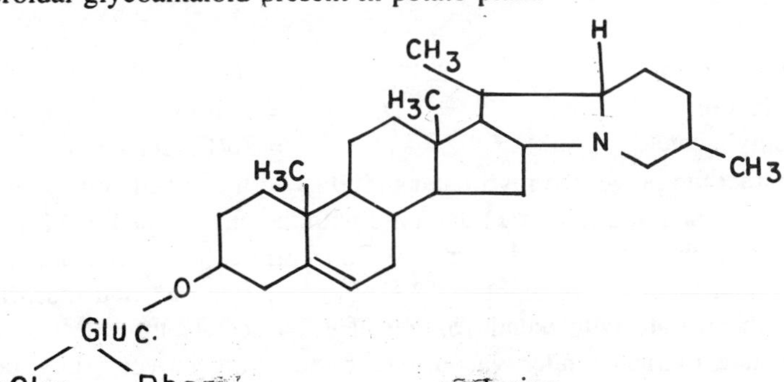

Solanine

Requirements:

Potatoes	= 500 g
Acetic acid (5x)	= 10 litres
Ammonium solution	= Sufficient amount
Methanol	= 50 ml

Procedure: Macerate the pieces of potatoes (500 g) with 5% acetic acid (10 litre) for 24 hours. Warm to 70°C, cool and adjust pH to 9.5 with ammonia solution. Centrifuge wash the precipitate with sufficient amount of 1% ammonia solution and centrifuge again. Discard the supernatant liquid and washings. Dry and weigh the residue. Purify it by dissolving in boiling methanol, filtering and concentrating until the glycoalkaloid starts to crystallize.

28. Isolation of Piperine from Black Pepper

Piperine is an alkaloid present in the fruits of *Piper nigrum* and other species of *Piper*.

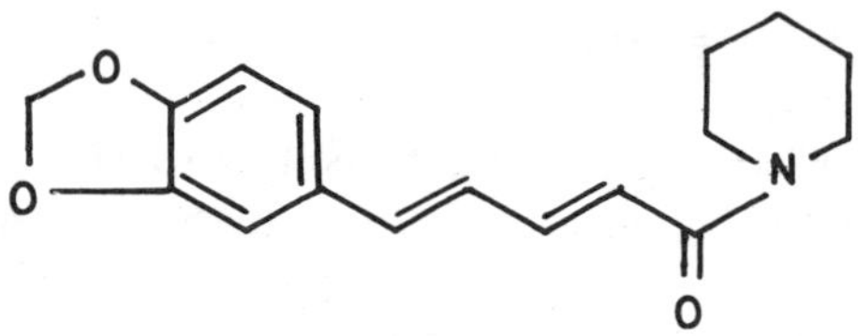

Piperine

Requirements:

Black Pepper	= 50 g
Ethanol (95%)	= 500 ml
Alcoholic KOH (10%)	= 50 ml

Procedure: Extract powdered drug (50 g) with ethanol (500 ml) in a Soxhlet apparatus for 3 hours. Filter the solution and concentrate under vacuum on a water bath. Add 10% alcoholic potassium hydroxide (50 ml) with constant stirring and filter. Allow the alcoholic solution to stand overnight. Piperine separates out as needles. The yield is about 2.5 per cent.

29. Isolation of Tannic Acid from Myrobalan

The fruits of *Terminalia Chebula* (Myrobalans) contain 20-30% tannins (ellagitannins).

Requirements:

Myrobalans	= 500 g
Alcohol	= 3 litres
Ethyl acetate	= Sufficient amount

Procedure: Extract the powdered myrobalans (500 g) with 95% ethanol (2 litres) on a shaker for 8 hours. Filter the extract and re-extract the marc with the ethanol (1 litre) for another 5 hours. Filter, wash and combine the filtrates and washings. Concentrate the extracts under vacuum. Dilute with distilled water and keep it overnight at 5° C. Filter the extract and discard the flocculent precipitate. Extract the filtrate with equal volume of ethyl acetate three times. Concentrate the combined ethyl acetate extracts under vacuum to remove the solvent. Dry tannic acid in a desiccator. The yield is about 14 per cent.

30. Isolation of Hecogenin from Agave (Sosal Leaves)

Hecogenin is a steroidal sapogenin (like diosgenin) used in the partial synthesis of cortisones and sex hormones. It is present in *Agave sisalanes* leaves.

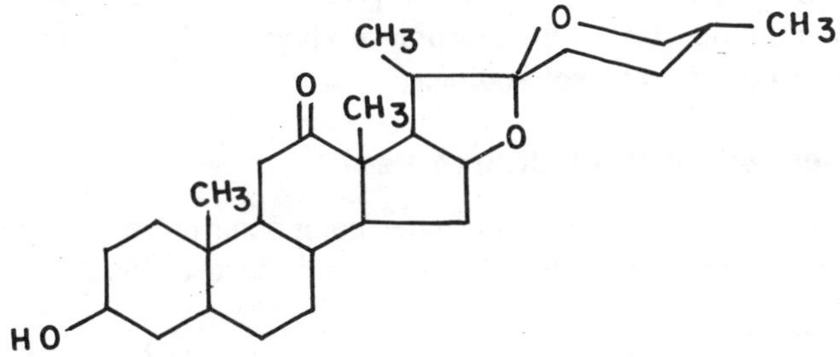

Requirements:

Sesal leaves	= 1 kg
Ethanol (20 %)	= 4 litres
Ethanolic HCl	= 400 ml
NaOH solution (5x)	= Sufficient amount
Ethanolic KOH (10%)	= 500 ml
Solvent ether	= 400 ml

Procedure: Extract air-dried, powdered leaves (1 kg) with 20% ethanol (4 litres) at about 100° for 12-16 hours. Filter the extract while hot and concentrate it under reduced pressure to get a sticky mass. Hydrolyze the residue with ethanolic hydrochloric acid (400 ml) at reflux temperature for 2 hours. Filter the reaction mixture and extract with solvent ether (3 × 100 ml). Wash the ether layer successively with water (3 × 50 ml), 5% aqueous sodium hydroxide (2 × 50 ml) and again with water (3 × 50 ml). Evaporate the ether extract and hydrolyze the residue again by refluxing with 10% alcoholic potassium hydroxide (400 ml) for 30 minutes. Extract the reaction mixture with solvent ether (3 × 150 ml). Distil off the ether extract. Dry the residue in a desiccator and weigh the final product.

31. Isolation of Solasodine from Berries of *Solanum khasianum*

Solasodine, a glycoalkaloid, is present in the berries of *Solanum khasianum* and *S. xanthocarpum* (family Solanaccae). It is used in the partial synthesis of corticosteroids.

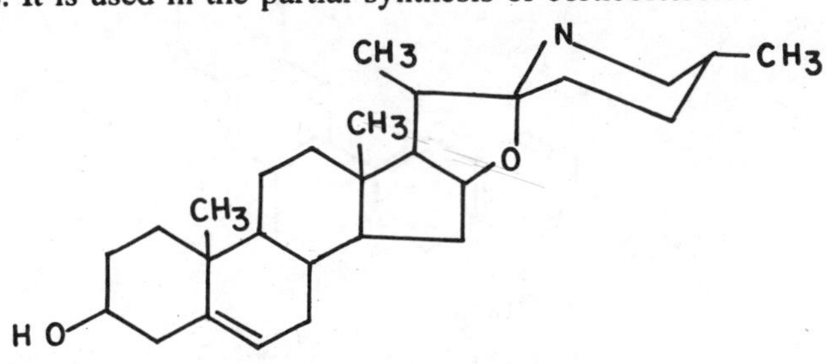

Requirements:

Plant material (berries)	= 100 g
Ethanol	= 500 ml
Conc. HCl	= 10 ml
Ammonia solution (10%)	= Sufficient ammount

Procedure: Extract dried and powdered plant material (100 g) with alcohol (500 ml) in a Soxhlet apparatus for 8 hours. Concentrate the extract to get a brown coloured viscous mass. Add concentrated hydrochloric acid (10 ml) and reflux the mixture for 4 hours. Cool the reaction mixture below 5°C for 6 hours and filter. To the precipitate add few ml of hot water and adjust pH 9 with ammonia solution. Reflux the reaction mixture for 2 hours, cool, filter the precipitate and dry to yield about 4% of crude solasodine.

32. Isolation of Hesperidin from Orange Peel

Hesperidin, a flavonoid compound, is a non-bitter compound present in the peels of orange and lemon. On hydrolysis it gives hesperetin, rhamnose and glucose. Hesperidin prevents fragitity of blood capillaries.

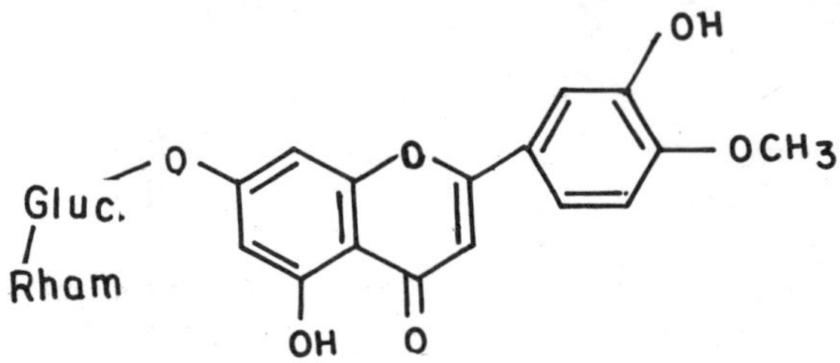

Requirements:

Orange peel	= 250 g
Petroleum ether	= 1 litre
Methanol	= 1 litre

Procedure: Reflux dried powdered orange peel (250 g) with light petroleum ether (1 litre) in a Soxhlet apparatus on a water bath for 1 hour. Filter the extract through a Buchner funnel and dry the merc at room temperature. Re-extract the powder with methanol (1 litre) in a Soxhlet apparatus for 3 hours. Concentrate the extract under reduced pressure to get a viscous mass. Dissolve the residue in dilute acetic acid solution and cool to crystallize hesperidin, m.p. 252-254°.

33. Isolation of Berberine from Berberis Roots

Berberine is present in the bark of roots or *Berberis lycium* and other species of *Berberis* (Family: Berberidaccae). It is used in the treatment of inflammatory conditions of mucous membrane.

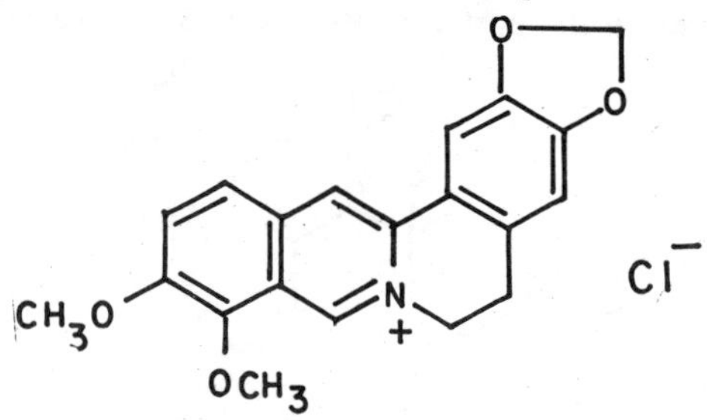

Berberine

Requirements:

Plant material	= 250 g
Ethanol	= 1 litre
Hydrochloric acid	= Sufficient amount
Acetone	= Sufficient amount

Procedure: Extract powdered roots (250 g) with ethanol (1 litre) in a Soxhlet apparatus for 12 hours. Distil off the solvent, dissolve the residue in sufficient amount of hot water and filter the hot solution to separate the resin. Excess of hydrochloric acid is added and kept for crystallization. The crystalline product was separated by filtration and recrystallized by dissolving in hot water and making the solution alkaline with a few drops of 10% sodium hydroxide solution. Add acetone to the solution and dilute it with equal volume of water. The mixture is cooled overnight at 5°C. The crystalline product is filtered off, and berberine-acetone dissolved in a mixture of alcohol and chloroform (10 : 1). Heat the solution to boiling and then cool at 5°C. The crystalline mass of berberine was filtered off.

34. Isolation of Sennosides as Calcium Salts from Senna Leaves

The leaves of *Cassia angustifolia* contain about 2.5% of total sennosides, calculated as sennoside B. These compounds are extracted as their calcium salts from the leaves and pods of Senna.

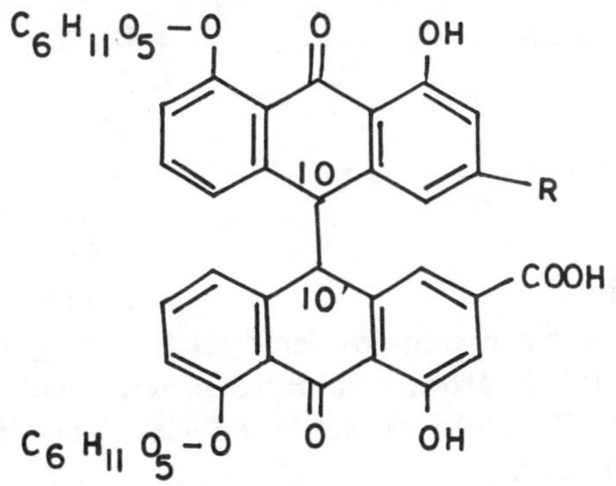

	R	10–10'
Sennoside A	COOH	trans
Sennoside B	COOH	meso
Sennoside C	CH_2OH	trans
Sennoside D	CH_2OH	meso

Requirements:

Senna leaves	= 250 g
Benzene	= 750 ml
Methanol (70%)	= 1.25 litre
Anhydrous calcium chloride	= 3 g

Procedure: Extract powdered leaves (250 g) with benzene (750 ml) for 2.5 hours in a Soxhlet apparatus. Concentrate the extract in vacuum to get a dark green viscous mass.

Dry the leaves left after benzene extraction in air and re-extract with 70% methanol (750 ml) on a shaker for 6 hours. Filter the extract and extract again the leaves with 70% methanol (500 ml) for 3 hours. Filter the solvent and combine the methanolic extracts. Concentrate the extract to 150 ml and acidify to pH 3.2 with hydrochloric acid with constant stirring. Cool the mixture for 2.5 hours at 5°C, filter in vacuum and add anhydrous calcium chloride (2.5 g in 35 ml alcohol) to the filtrate with stirring. Adjust pH of the solution to 8 with ammonia solution and set aside for 2.5 hours. Filter the solution in vacuum and dry the precipitate in a desiccator containing phosphorus pentoxide.

35. Isolation of Strychnine and Brucine from Nux Vomica Seeds

The seeds of nux vomica contain about 2-5% of strychnine and brucine.

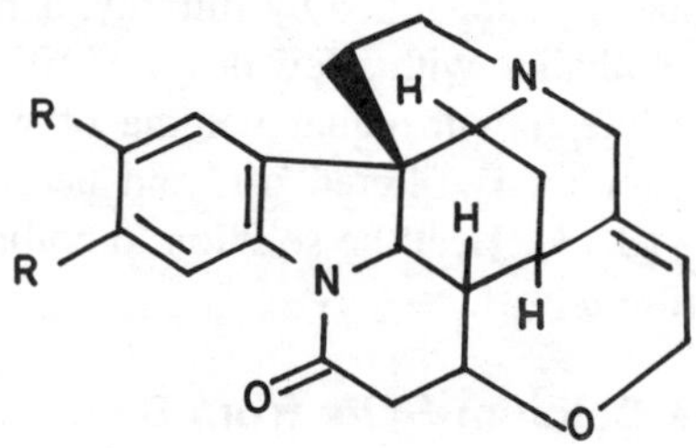

Brucine (R = OCH_3)
Strychnine (R = H)

Requirements:

Nux vomica seeds	= 100 g
Slaked lime	= 10 g
Chloroform	= 500 ml
Ammonia soslution	= Sufficient amount
Ethanol	= Sufficient amount
Oxalic acid	= Sufficient amount
Dilute H_2SO_4	= 150 ml

Procedure: Prepare a paste by mixing powdered seeds (100 g) with slaked lime (10 g) by addition of water and dry it 100°C. Extract the dried material with chloroform (500 ml) in a Soxhlet apparatus for 6 hours. Shake the extract thrice with dilute sulphuric acid (4 × 50 ml). Combine the acid extracts and filter.

Add excess of ammonia to the acid extract to precipitate the alkaloids. Dissolve the precipitate in ethanol 25%) to isolate brucine. Filter off undissolved strychnine and purify by repeated crystallization from ethanol.

Concentrate the filtrate and precipitate brucine as oxalate by neutralization with oxalic acid solution. Wash the precipitate with cold ethanol, dissolve in minimum amount of hot water decolourize with animal charcoal, filter and dry the filtrate. Dissolve the residue with small amount of acetone and evaporate the solvent to give brucine oxalate.

14

Reagents and Solutions

Acetic Acid, Dilute : Contains approximately 6% w/v of CH_3COOH. Dilute glacial acetic acid (57 ml) to 1000 ml with water.

Ammonia- Ammonium Chloride Solution Strong : Dissolve ammonium chloride (67.5 g) in strong ammonia solution (740 ml) and add sufficient water to produce 1000 ml.

Ammonia Solution, Dilute : Dilute strong ammonia solution (425 ml) to 1000 ml with water.

Ammonium Acetate Solution : Dissolve ammonium acetate (150 g) in water (200 ml). Add glacial acetic acid (3 ml) and dilute to 1000 ml with water.

Anisaldehyde-Acetic Acid Reagent : Anisaldehyde (0.5 ml) is mixed with 98% acetic acid (10 ml).

Anisaldehyde-Sulphuric Acid Reagent : Anisaldehyde (0.5 ml) is mixed with glacial acetic acid (10 ml), followed by methanol (85 ml) and concentrated sulphuric acid (5 ml).

Antimony (III) Chloride Reagent : 20% solution of antimony. (III) chloride in chloroform.

Barfoeds Reagent : Dissolve crystalline copper acetate (6.5 g) in 1% acetic acid solution (100 ml).

Barium Chloride : A 10% w/v solution of barium chloride in water.

Benedict's Solution : Dissolve crystalline copper sulphate (1.73 g) in water (100 ml) and add to it a solution of sodium citrate (17.3 g) and anhydrous Na_2CO_3 (10 g) in H_2O (80 ml). Dilute the solution to 100 ml with water.

Benzidine Reagent : Benzidine (0.5 g) is dissolved in glacial acetic acid (10 ml)-and the volume adjusted to 100 ml with ethanol.

Bromine Solution: Dissolve bromine (9.6 ml) and potassium bromide (30 g) in sufficient water to produce 100 ml.

Ceric Ammonium Sulphate : Ceric sulphate (1 g) is soaked in water (40 ml). Add trichloroacetic acid (10 g), slowly add drop by drop sulphuric acid (d 1.84), until the solution clarifies.

Chlorinated Lime Solution: Mix chlorinated lime (100 g) with water (1000 ml), transfer the mixture to a stoppered bottle, set aside for three hours, shaking occasionally and filter through calico.

Chlorinated lime must be prepared freshly.

Dragendorff's Reagent : (A) Bismuth carbonate (2.6 g) and sodium iodide (7.0 g) are boiled for few minute with glacial acetic acid (25 ml). After 12 hours, the precipitated sodium acetate crystals are filtered off 20 ml of the clear, red-brown filtrate is mixed with ethyl acetate (8 ml) and stored in a brown bottle.

(B) Basic bismuth nitrate (0.85 g) is dissolved in water (40 ml) and glacial acetic acid

(10 ml) followed by addition of potassium iodide (8 g) dissolved in water (20 ml).

2, 4-Dinitrophenylhydrazine : Dissolve 2, 4-dinitrophenylhydrazine (2 g) in concentrated sulphuric acid (10 ml). Add sufficient alcohol to produce 200 ml.

2, 6-Dichlorophenolindophenol Solution: Warm 2, 6-dichlorophenolindophenol sodium salt (0.1 g) with water (100 ml) and filter.

Diphenylcarbazide : A 0.2% w/v solution of diphenylcarbazide in a mixture of glacial acetic acid (10 ml) and alcohol (90 ml).

Fehling Solution A: Dissolve crystalline copper sulphate (34.64 g) in water (500 ml) containing a few drops of concentrated sulphuric acid.

Fehling Solution B: Dissolve sodium potassium tartrate (Rochelle salt) (173 g) and sodium hydroxide (60 g) in water and made the solution to 500 ml with water.

Ferric Chloride Test Solution : A 10% w/v solution of ferric chloride (10 g) in water (100 ml).

Iodine Solution : Dissolve iodine (2 g) and potassium iodide (3 g) in water to produce 100 ml.

Kedde Reagent : Freshly prepared ethanolic 3, 5-dinitrobenzoic acid solution (5 ml) are mixed with 2M sodium hydroxide solution (5 ml).

Lead Acetate Solution : A 10% w/v solution of lead acetate (10 g) in carbon dioxide free water (100 ml).

Liebermann-Burchard Reagent : Acetic anhydride (5 ml) and concentrated sulphuric acid (5 ml) are added carefully to absolute alcohol (5 ml), while cooling in ice. The reagent must be freshly prepared.

Magnesium Uranyl Acetate Solution : Heat on a water bath uranyl acetate (3-2 g), magnesium acetate (10 g), glacial acetic acid (2 ml) and water (30 ml). When the solution is complete, allow to cool, add alcohol (50 ml) and dilute with water (100 ml). Allow to stand for twenty four hours and filter.

Mercuric Acetate Solution : A 5% solution of mercuric acetate (5 g) in glacial acetic acid (100 ml).

Mercury Nitrate Solution (Millon's Reagent) : Dissolve mercury (3 ml) in cold fuming nitric acid (27 ml), dilute the solution with equal volume of water.

Molisch's Regent : Dissolve α-naphthol (10 g) in rectified spirit (100 ml).

Ninhydrin Reagent : Ninhydrin (30 mg) are dissolved in n-butanol (10 ml), followed by 98% of acetic acid (0.3 ml).

Perchloric acid : 2% aqueous perchloric acid.

Phloroglucinol Solution : A 1% solution in 90% ethanol with hydrochloric acid for staining lignin.

Phosphomolybdic Acid Reagent : 20% Ethanolic solution of phosphomolybdic acid.

Phenylhydrazine Solution : Dissolve phenylhydrazine hydrochloride (65 g) previously recrystallized from aqueous alcohol in sufficient of a mixture of sulphuric acid (70 ml) and water (30 ml) to produce 100 ml.

Picric Acid Solution : A 1% w/v solution of picric acid in hot water (100 ml)..

Potassium Ferricyanide Solution : Wash about potassium ferricyanide crystals (1 g) with a small amount of water and dissolve the warhed crystals in water (100 ml).

Potassium Ferrocyanide Solution : A 5% w/v solution of potassium ferrocyanide in water (100 ml).

Potassium Mercuri-iodide Solution (Mayer's Reagent): Add mercuric chloride (1.36 g) dissolved in water (60 ml) to a solution of potassium iodide (5 g) in water (20 ml), mix and add sufficient water to produce 100 ml.

Potassium Mercuri-iodide Solution, (Alkaline Nessler Reagent) : To potassium iodide (3.5 g), add mercuric chloride (1.25 g) dissolved in water (80 ml), add cold saturated solution of mercuric chloride in water with constant stirring until a slight red precipitate remains. Dissolve sodium hydroxide (12 g) in the solution, add a little more of the cold saturated solution of mercuric chloride and sufficient water to produce 100 ml. Allow to stand and decant the clear liquid.

Potassium Permanganate Solution (Baeyer's Reagent)

Dissolve potassium permanganate (1 g) in water (100 ml) and add few drops of potassium hydroxide solution to have a clear solution of pink colour.

Pyridine Bromide Solution : Dissolve pyridine (10 ml) and sulphuric acid (5.4 ml) in glacial acetic acid (20 ml) keeping the mixture cool. Add bromine (2-6 ml) dissolved in glacial acetic acid (20 ml) and dilute with glacial acetic acid to 100 ml.

Pyridine bromide solution should be freshly prepared.

Phenolphthalein Solution : Dissolve 5 g in 50% alcohol (500 ml).

Schiff's Reagent : Pass sulphur dioxide gas in 1% solution of rosanaline till its colour is discharged. Filter and store the solution in a tightly stoppered bottle.

Silver Nitrate Solution : A 5% w/v solution of silver nitrate in water.

Sodium Bisulphite Solution : Dissolve sodium bisulphite (10 g) in sufficient water to make 30 ml.

Sodium Cobaltinitrite Solution : A 30% w/v solution of sodium cobaltinitrite is water (100 ml).

Sodium Nitroprusside Solution : A 1% w/v solution of sodium nittoprusside in water (100 ml).

Stannous Chloride Solution : Dissolve stannous chloride (30 g) in hydrochloric acid (100 ml) and add sufficient water to produce 1000 ml.

Sudan III Solution : It is a solution in equal parts of glycerin and alcohol. It stains oils and suberized walls.

Tannic Acid Solution : A 10% w/v solution of tannic acid in water (100 ml).

Thioacetamide Reagent : Add 1 ml of a mixture of N sodium hydroxide (15 ml), water (5 ml) and glycerin (20 ml) to a 4% w/v solution of thioacetamide (0.2 ml) in water. Heat on water bath for twenty seconds and cool.

Thioacetamide reagent should be prepared immediately before use.

Vanillin-Hydrochloric Acid Reagent : Vanillin (1 g) is dissolved in ethanol (100 ml) and concentrated hydrochloric acid (3 ml) is added.

Vanillin-Sulphuric Acid Reagent : Vanillin (3 g) is dissolved in ethanol (100 ml) and concentrated sulphuric acid (1 ml) added.

Appendix I

Recording of Volumetric Analysis

Object : Perform the assay of sodium carbonate.

Reference : I.P. 1985 Page A-226.

Standard Limit : It contains not less than 99% and not more than the equivalent of 105.0% of $Na_2CO_3.10H_2O$.

Reactions and Theory : Sodium carbonate is the salt of a strong base and weak acid. The aqueous solution is alkaline due to hydrolysis.

It is assayed by titration will 0.5 N H_2SO_4 using bromophenol blue as an indicator.

$$Na_2CO_3 + H_2SO_4 \longrightarrow Na_2SO_4 + CO_2 + H_2O$$

Equivalent Factor : Each ml of 0.5N H_2SO_4 is equivalent to 0.07154 g of $Na_2CO_3.\ 10H_2O$.

Colour Change at End Point : At the end point there is acidic pH. Hence a blue colour is changed into yellow colour.

Procedure : Weigh sodium carbonate (2 g), dissolve in water (20 ml) and titrate it with 0.5N H_2SO_4 using bromophenol blue solution as an indicator.

Observation and Calculation

S.No.	Initial Volume of 0.5 H_2SO_4 Solution (ml)	Final Volume of 0.5 H_2SO_4 Solution (ml)	Value of 0.5 H_2SO_4 Consumed (V. ml)
1.			
2.			
3.			

Calculation

$$\text{Percentage purity : } \frac{V \times N \times 0.07154}{0.5 \times W} \times 1000$$

V = Volume of 0.5 N H_2SO_4 solution.

N = Normality of the sulphuric acid.

W = Weight of the sodium carbonate.

Result : The percentage purity of given sample of $Na_2\ CO_3\ 10\ H_2O$ is ....

Appendix II

Recording of Qualitative Organic Analysis

Object : Identify the given organic compound.

Procedure

S. No.	*Experiment*	*Observation*	*Inference*
Preliminary tests			
1.	Physical Properties		
	(i) Physical state	Liquid	
	(ii) Colour	White	
	(iii) Smell	No specific smell	Nitro-compounds absent
	(iv) Solubility	Soluble in hot water	May be aromatic compound.
2.	Ignition test	The compound burns with smoky flame	May be aromatic compound.
Detection of Elements			
3.	$FeSO_4$ test Sodium extract + $FeSO_4$ + boil + dil. H_2SO_4	No prussian blue or greenish blue colour	Nitrogen absent
4.	Nitroprusside test Sodium extract + Sodium nitroprusside	No violet or purple colour	Sulphur absent
5.	Silver nitrate test Sodium extract + dil HNO_3 + $AgNO_3$ solution	No precipitate (chlorine, bromine, iodine absent)	Halogens absent

Tests for Functional Groups

Since nitrogen, sulphur and halogens are absent, therefore the functional groups corresponding to these elements are absent and functional groups corresponding to oxygen and hydrogen are present (i.e. COOH, — CHO, C = O, OH, carbohydrate and hydrocarbon).

S. No.	*Experiment*	*ObservationInference*
6. Blue litmus paper test Organic compound + blue litmus	It turned red	—COOH group is present
7. $NaHCO_3$ test organic compound + $NaHCO_3$ solution	Brisk efferves-cences occur	—COOH group is present
8. Determine the m.p.	121°C	may be benzoic acid

From the above inference, the compound is an aromatic acid with m.p.. 121°. Examine the list of compounds. The compound is probable benzoic acid

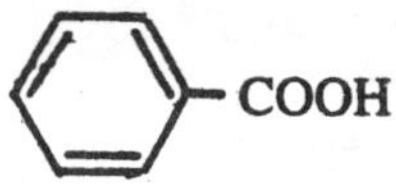

Confirmatory Tests and Derivatives

S. No.	*Experiment*	*Observation Inference*
9. Ester formation test Organic compound + ethyl alcohol + 1–2 drops conc. H_2SO_4 + heat	Fruity odour present	benzoic acid
10. Nitration Organic compound + conc. HNO_3 + conc. H_2SO_4 + shake and warm for 5 minutes and pour into water	yellow solid separates out	benzoic acid present
11. $FeCl_3$ test Neutral aqueous solution of the organic compound + neutral solution of $FeCl_3$	Buff precipitate	benzoic acid is present
12.. Derivative formation Yellow solid obtained on nitration is filtered, washed, dried and the m.p. is determined.	m.p. 140°	m.p. of m-nitro-benzoic acid is 140° (literature)

Result : The given organic compound is found to be benzoic acid.

Index